Care of the Older Adult

7835708

Joan Carson Breitung, RN, MA

Director, Practical Nursing Program,
Roger L. Putnam Vocational Technical High School,
Springfield, Massachusetts

The Tiresias Press, Inc.
New York City

Library of Congress Catalog Card Number: 80-51870
International Standard Book Number: 0-913292-05-2

Printed in U.S.A.

Current printing (last digit) 10 9 8 7 6 5 4 3 2 1

Cover photo courtesy of Skippy Gurau.

Line drawings are by Yumi Izumito and Margery R. Frank.

Credits

We wish to thank the following persons and companies for the use of their material: The American Hospital Association; Ames Company, a Division of Miles Laboratories, Inc.; Baystate Medical Center, Springfield, Massachusetts; Boehringer Ingelheim Ltd.; Campbell Soup Company; Charles Carson,; Skippy Gurau, Jewish Home of Western Massachusetts; J.B. Lippincott Company for material from *Textbook of Medical-Surgical Nursing,* 3rd edition, by Brunner and Suddarth; *Los Angeles Times;* Lumex, Inc.; Ed Malley; Mercy Hospital, Springfield, Massachusetts; Monoject,Division of Sherwood Medical; C. V. Mosby Company and Catherine Parker Anthony for material from Mrs. Anthony's *Structures and Functions of the Body;* National Technical Institute for the Deaf; W.B. Saunders Company and Audrey Sutton for material from Mrs. Sutton's *Basic Bedside Nursing Techniques;* Thomas G. Ferguson Associates, Inc., and Bard Urological Division; United, Division of Howmedica, Inc.; and The Upjohn Company. Credits are also listed with these materials.

Care of the Older Adult

Dedication

To the elderly, who deserve nursing care that is given with skill and sensitivity.

Contents

Preface

The purpose of this book is to encourage productive and meaningful nursing care of the most rapidly increasing segment of our population—adults over 65. In 1900 they made up four percent of the population. Today the figure is between 11 and 12 percent. Fifty years from now it is expected to rise to 20 percent. Some of us will be part of that population.

Care of the Older Adult was written primarily for practical nurses, but many others, including registered nurses, nursing assistants, and home health aides, will find it useful. Social workers, psychologists, and directors of day care and senior citizen centers will find the book to be a reliable and serviceable guide for understanding the various physical and mental disabilities that many of the aged incur. For those who are themselves elderly (and their families), the sections on choosing a nursing home, retirement, day care, nutrition, and alternate modes of living will be of particular interest. Instructors in courses on geriatrics and gerontology will discover that the book is a versatile teaching tool.

Part One introduces the student to geriatrics, explores the myths and facts of aging, discusses nursing home placement and alternatives to placement, examines the mental disorders of old age, promotes an understanding of the mental anguish of aphasia, deals with incontinence and constipation, and contains a chapter on sexuality and aging. It also contains a chapter on nutrition with a recent survey by the author on the nutritional practices of the well adult over 65.

The book is unique not only for its range of subject matter but for the way in which the nine chapters on the body systems (Part Two) are presented. For each body system, the book:

- reviews in simple terms the anatomy of the system
- describes the age-related changes that can occur
- gives related nursing procedures

It is hoped that this book will contribute to an understanding of the aging process and that it will encourage superior care that will add to the health and comfort of our elders.

—Joan Breitung

Acknowledgments

I would like to acknowledge the following people for their help and suggestions while I was preparing this book:

Grace Breitung
Nancy Callahan
Charles Carson
Daniel Carson
Mary Carson
Virginia Carson
Gladys Chernock
James Clune
Mary Conway
Anna Cousins
Mary Lou DiGiacomo
Eileen Donoghue
Margery Frank
Nancy Gilbert
Kathryn Gillispie
Carolyn Gove

Skippy Gurau
Florence Gurvitch
Anna Hoffman
Yumi Izumito
Marguerite Johnson
Terry La Plante
Clara Lepow
Madlyn McNiff
Dorothy Mozden
Eileen Neville
David and Ruth Nirenstein
Stan Sherer
Dan Trombler
Ralph Wener
Maureen Wark
Dorothy Zoeller

Special thanks to my patient and understanding family: my husband, Ben, and my children, Eve, Evan, Benedict, Anne, Joan, Claire, Erik, and Barbara.

PART I

The Many Aspects of Aging

Even the oldest tree some fruit may bear
. . . For age is opportunity no less
Than youth itself, though in another dress.

—Longfellow

1

Introduction to Aging

Objectives

After completing this chapter, the student should be able to:

- separate the myths from the facts of aging
- take a geriatric patient's nursing history
- understand the importance of a nursing care plan for elderly patients

While there was a birth of interest in the causes and effects of aging about 30 years ago, many of us still participate in or contribute to that well-entrenched prejudice, ageism. Ageism is a bias against the elderly, derived from the American attitude that what is important and desirable is youth. In *Aging and Mental Health*, Butler and Lewis state that "Prejudice toward the elderly is an attempt by younger generations to shield themselves from the fact of their own eventual aging and death and to avoid having to deal with the social and economic problems of increasing numbers of older people."

Have you ever observed patronizing behavior by health care professionals toward old people? Step onto any medical/surgical floor in an acute care hospital and you'll see tolerant smiles or hear amusing anecdotes as staff members discuss a geriatric patient. Often you will observe a pessimistic attitude toward the treatment of elderly admissions—"Why bother with all these tests and drugs for someone 80 years old?" Visit virtually any nursing home and you'll see old ladies made "cute" with pigtails and hairbows, and hear condescending responses (and some irritable responses) by staff members to confused and disoriented residents.

Attitudes and behaviors change slowly, but they do change. Health care personnel are becoming increasingly involved in meeting the physical and emotional needs of old people. Care is not restricted to long term facilities, either. The elderly seeking treatment are seen in acute care hospitals, physicians' offices, and outpatient clinics. Many enjoy the benefits of day care centers.

Education, empathy, and enthusiasm are qualities that will promote superior geriatric nursing. It's a demanding discipline but an extremely satisfying one.

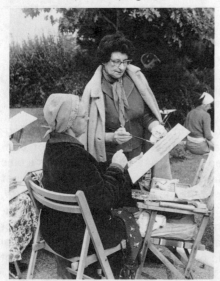

Older American instructing an art class.   Courtesy of Charles Carson.

Myths And Facts

There are many myths about aged adults. Read the following examples and see if you have ever confused a myth with a fact.

Myth: Old people are sickly and most of them are hospitalized.

Fact: Less than five percent of the elderly are confined to institutions. Although more than 80 percent of them have some type of chronic health problem, ranging from arthritis to vascular disease, yet, despite this, better than 80 percent are up and taking care of themselves. This popular myth may have grown from the fact that between two-thirds and three-fourths of hospital admissions are over the age of 65.

Myth: The poor can tolerate the impact of aging better than the affluent because the poor have never had anything anyway.

Fact: As the poor become elderly their problems intensify. Many live in substandard housing. The necessities of life, i.e., food, shelter, and medical expenses, become discouragingly expensive to poor people. This has given rise to the next myth.

Myth: Elderly people don't need to spend much money for clothing, recreation, transportation, and so on.

Fact: They would like very much to spend money on these things, but the poor among them just can't afford to. The director of a Golden Age center made this revealing comment: "Today, there's barely a dress code anywhere. You may go where you wish and dress as you please. Anything goes. But these people [indicating the members] were raised in a generation where you *dressed* to go out. Not having what they consider 'suitable' clothes or enough changes of clothes often keeps many of our members from participating here."

Myth: The blue collar worker has a difficult adjustment to retirement.

Fact: No doubt some blue collar workers view retirement with concern, but many have good pensions and retirement benefits. In addition, they have worked regular hours for many years and have had time to find outside interests and hobbies. This is in marked contrast to the professional man who has committed all his time and attention to his career and faces retirement with nothing to take its place.

Myth: Old people are senile.

Fact: This is unkind stereotyping of the elderly when they exhibit forgetfulness, memory lapses, confusion, or slow reactions. Unfortunately, the term "senility" is used by lay persons and professionals alike and this indiscriminate labeling often postpones or clouds the diagnosis of treatable conditions. When any one of the above-mentioned conditions happens to younger people, we shrug it off. If it persists, we become concerned and seek treatment. But when the person is 65 or older, it is easier to use the catchall term "senility."

Checking What You Know

One way to begin the study of new material is to determine what you already know. Complete the following True-False quiz by circling T or F and then check your answers on page 20.

T   F   1. Life expectancy has increased through modern medical advances.

T   F   2. Elderly people need at least eight hours of sleep each night.

T   F   3. A small percentage (five percent or less) of the elderly are institutionalized.

T   F   4. For the adult past 65, chronological age and biological age are the same.

T   F   5. Depression is quickly diagnosed in adults over 65.

T   F   6. Senile patients escape depression because they are not in touch with reality.

T   F   7. If the blood supply to the brain is impaired, the resulting damage to the brain is always irreversible.

T   F   8. There is a definite decrease in the short-term memory of adults over 65.

T   F   9. Elderly people do not tolerate pain well.

T   F 10. People need information about the sexual needs of the elderly.

T   F   11. Reminiscing is helpful in adapting to the aging process.

T   F   12. Listening to elderly people is an effective way to learn about geriatrics and gerontology.

The Nursing History

When a patient is admitted to a long term facility, a nursing history should be taken and a nursing care plan should be made.

The nursing history collects data in a structured, organized way. It should be flexible and should be designed to illustrate the needs of the patient and to fit the requirements of the particular health care agency that admits the patient. It is helpful if the family can also be interviewed. If the patient is brain damaged or comatose and no family cooperation can be obtained, no history is taken.

It isn't always easy to gather information for a nursing history from an elderly person. It requires sensitivity and good communication skills on the part of the interviewer, especially if the patient cannot hear well. About 25 percent of persons over 65 have some hearing impairment. In such cases, the interviewer should position herself so that the person being questioned can see her lips and eyes. If the patient is profoundly deaf, it may be necessary to resort to writing.

The interviewer should be aware that a patient's vocabulary may not be the same as hers. If the interviewer asks, "How often do you void?" the patient may look at her blankly. "How often do you urinate or pass water?" may be language more suitable for some individuals.

When discussing medications, be sure that the patient understands that these include over-the-counter drugs as well as prescriptions.

Gathering data is an important first step in developing effective plans of care, but some questions may be interpreted as intrusive. Avoid making the patient feel uncomfortable. Allow enough time to gain the patient's confidence. After all, the questions can be postponed for a while, and can even be asked informally while assisting the patient with the activities of daily living.

Sample Nursing History Form *

1.   Vital statistics
      Name _____ Age____ Sex: □F □M
      Marital Status _____Social Security Number_____
      Residence_____ Telephone_____
      Whom to call in an emergency_____
      Physician_____Telephone _____
      Medical diagnosis _____
      Blood type _____ Allergies _____

2.   General appearance
      Height_____ Weight_____
      Grooming (hair, makeup, clothing) _____
      _____
      Position (posture) _____

3.   Patient's understanding of illness
      State why patient believes he/she is in the facility _____
      _____
      Describe the events in the patient's life about the time he/she notic-
      ed indications of illness _____
      _____
      Describe how patient's life has been affected by illness _____
      _____

4.   Patient's expectations
      Describe what patient expects to happen while he/she is in the
      facility _____
      Describe patient's expectations regarding the nursing staff _____
      _____

5.   Social and cultural history
      Occupation _____
      Educational background (level achieved) _____
      Languages spoken _____
      Members of patient's immediate family _____
      _____

6.   Significant data
      Rest and sleep patterns:
          Usual bedtime _____ Measures to induce sleep _____
          _____Sleep pattern in terms of falling asleep

and then awakening during the night _____
Number of pillows used _____
Elimination:
  Frequency_____ Time(s) _____ Problems _____
Breathing:
  Rate_____ Rhythm _____ Ease of respirations __
Nutrition:
  Likes _____ Dislikes _____
  Self-feed?_____ Religious restrictions _____
  Dentures _____ Swallowing ability _____ Anorexia _____
Skin:
  Color_____ Turgor _____ Texture _____
  Eruptions _____ Bruises _____ Decubiti _____
  Wounds _____ Odor _____
Activity:
  Gait _____ Range of motion _____
  Activities of daily living _____
  Needs help with ADL _____ Sexuality needs and patterns _____
  _____
Recreation: (Favorite diversions, sports, TV, hobbies, reading mat-
ter, etc.) _____
Communication:
  Verbal behavior (coherent, confused, etc.) _____
Temperament (describe what makes the patient happy, unhappy):
_____
Senses (impaired sight, hearing, right- or left-handedness, pro-
stheses) _____

7. Describe what is important to the patient. State what helps him/her
    feel secure, comfortable, safe: _____
    _____

8. Nursing diagnosis, goals, and orders: _____
    _____
    _____

_____

* This suggested outline for a nursing history was adapted from the University of
Florida Nursing History Form.

Nursing Care Plans

Most hospitals and long term care facilities have nursing care plans. These are designs for the patient's care based on a summary of the patient's problems, suggested approaches to the problems, and an evaluation of the action to be taken. The nursing team, the patient's family, and sometimes various resource persons (dietitians, physical therapists, and so on) contribute to the care plan. The physician is chiefly concerned with the patient's medical diagnosis and treatment, although often he or she is an important resource person.

Nursing care plans should be dynamic and constantly changing to meet the changing needs of the patient. While every health care agency has a different method of maintaining care plans (kardexes and looseleaf books are often used), they all share one common problem: keeping the plans up to date. Staff has to be encouraged to revise the nursing care plans whenever necessary. This can be done daily or at the end of each shift.

Communicating With the Elderly

The following quotation* expresses a sensible approach to dealing with elderly patients that can be used not only by physicians but by everyone, especially nurses.

"It is quite common to find fear of aging and fear of death among members of our youth-oriented society. The recognition of such fears . . . is of utmost importance in establishing effective communication with the elderly.

"The physician must attempt to separate myths about aging from reality. For example, the . . . elderly are especially sensitive to being labeled 'senile,' 'mentally ill,' or 'hypochondriac.' The physician should try to empathize with the elderly patient. Putting yourself in the other person's shoes is an ability not easily taught by textbooks and can only be learned through personal experiences.

* *Blazer, Dan. "Techniques for Communicating with Your Elderly Patient."* Geriatrics, *p. 79, November, 1978.*

"Approach the elderly patient with respect . . . . try to approach the patient from the front. Greet the patient by surname rather than by given name unless he or she wishes to be addressed by a given name.

"Pay attention to nonverbal communication. Be alert for changes in facial expressions, gestures, postures. These nonverbal signs can provide considerable information about conditions such as depression or anxiety. Touch may also be an effective way to relax and make contact with the elderly patient. As a rule, the elderly are less inhibited about physical touch. Holding the patient's hand or resting your hand on his arm may be very reassuring.

"Be realistic but hopeful. Physicians who work with the elderly often deny the problems of late life. But neither the physician nor the patient believes the phrases like 'You'll live to be 100,' or, 'It's nothing to worry about,' and the physician should avoid using them. He should never abandon all hope for the patient . . . but he should work in the here and now."

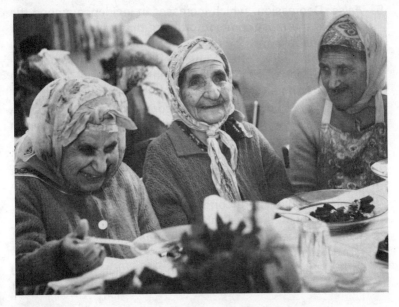

Three sisters enjoy a family gathering in Italy. Courtesy of Skippy Gurau.

Answers to the Self-Check on Page 14

1. *True.* Life expectancy has been increased through modern medical advances. In 1900, life expectancy was 43 years. In 1920, it was 54 for men and 55 for women. In 1950, it was 66 for men and 72 for women. In 1978, it was 67 for men and 74 for women.

2. *False.* Aged individuals may need more *rest,* but they actually need less sleep. Five to seven hours a night is sufficient.

3. *True.* Very few of the total population of elderly persons are institutionalized. About 80 percent live in their own homes. Another 14 or 15 percent live with relatives.

4. *False.* When we speak about biological aging we are talking about cellular life. Chronological age means age in years. No two people age the same biologically, and different rates and degrees of aging can be found in the same age group. Also, one body system can deteriorate with age (the skin, for instance) while there is almost no change in the other systems.

5. *False.* Depression, which increases in incidence among the aged, is the most common problem that psychiatrists treat elderly people for. It is difficult to diagnose because the symptoms are often obscured by stereotypical behaviors—lack of vitality, sluggishness, brooding—which are thought to be an inevitable part of growing old.

6. *False.* Senile patients can become depressed. In fact, sometimes it's depression, not chronic brain syndrome (or organic brain syndrome), that provokes symptoms of senility.

7. *False.* Certain medical problems can be treated and thus improve the blood supply to the brain. Examples of such medical problems are congestive heart failure and dehydration with resulting electrolyte imbalance.

8. *True.* Short-term memory does decrease with age, but long-term memory is rarely impaired.

9. *False.* Elderly people tolerate pain quite well. It's not a good thing, though, because some complaints that they shrug off

as due to "old age" should be investigated before they develop into something serious. Peripheral pain sensations are reduced and this can be harmful as in cases of heating pad burns, scalding, and so on.

10. *True.* Sexual information is necessary for the aged so that they can avoid feeling guilty about sexual feelings, and it is necessary for the younger members of society so that they will recognize that the sexual experiences of the aged are natural and good.

11. *True.* Reminiscing is important and can be therapeutic for elderly people. Memories are sometimes all old people have to remind them that they were once vital contributors to society.

12. *True.* By listening to old people, you can begin to appreciate many of the changes that take place in the elderly—impaired hearing, short-term memory loss, slowed reaction time, and others.

2

The Nursing Home
and Its Alternatives

Objectives

After completing this chapter, the student should be able to:
- understand how geriatric discharge planning can be improved through the use of proper resource agencies
- list the alternatives to nursing home placement that may be available to qualified people
- understand the need that families who must place their relative in a nursing home have for support and counseling
- explain how to choose a nursing home
- explain the four levels of care that long term facilities offer
- tell patients and their families what the rights of patients are
- evaluate the strengths and weaknesses of nursing home ombudsmen programs

The staff in acute care hospitals is commonly unaware of the strong psychological impact that sudden disability has on elderly patients. Staff members are used to fast turnover. They don't welcome changing a busy medical/surgical floor into a geriatric unit and, moreover, they are too busy to coax elderly patients to eat or to listen to faltering conversations. Once the acute problem (the admitting diagnosis) is solved, the discharge procedure is set in motion. But discharge where? To what? If hospitalization is traumatic for elderly adults, even more traumatic is nursing home placement afterwards. How can adjustment be eased?

Alternatives to Nursing Homes

To force the elderly into institutions when there are reasonable alternatives is a monumental disaster. Those responsible for discharge planning should, where feasible, consider the alternatives of home care and group living.

Home Care

Many aged persons, even those with multiple chronic illnesses, can be given adequate care in their own homes. Home Care Corporation is a nonprofit, private agency that plans, coordinates, and contracts for the home care of adults over 60. The various services are funded through Titles III and VII of the Older Americans Act and Title XX of the Social Security Act as well as city, town, and community organizations. Local Councils on the Aging can direct inquirers for supportive services to available agencies.

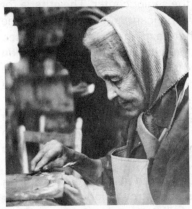

Learning a new skill (ceramics) at 87. Courtesy of Skippy Gurau.

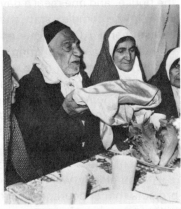

A seder (a religiously-oriented Jewish meal) in Israel.   Courtesy of Skippy Gurau.

Some of the services offered are: health screening, homemaking (light housekeeping and meal preparation), chore service (heavy duty household work), mental health, and legal services. Most of these services are free, while others have a nominal fee set on a sliding scale.

Congregate Housing and Communal Living

Another alternative to premature and/or inappropriate nursing home placement is group living, either in congregate housing or communal living quarters.

Congregate housing is sheltered housing for elderly and/or handicapped adults. A residential complex is modified to accommodate their needs by installing wide doorways, ramps, low cabinets, and so forth. There is a security guard and often a physician or nurse is on call for health emergencies.

Communal living simply means that a group of people live together and share expenses. Jon A. Larkin, executive director of the Wilmington (Delaware) Senior Center, described an experiment in communal living in *Perspective on Aging.* A family of nine unrelated elderly persons live in a large, three-bathroom duplex. Each resident pays a nominal rent, which entitles him or her to a private bedroom and shared kitchen, living room, sitting room, and bathroom. The rent also includes utilities, two meals a day at the house, and one meal a day at the senior center. The criteria for living in the complex state that an applicant must have an income of less than $7,000 a year and that he or she must be committed to the experiment of sharing a home with other people. Mr. Larkin states: "Those who have worked to develop Brandywine House believe there is great potential for the same or similar alternative living arrangements for older persons:

"Cities can use boarded-up housing for a useful purpose — while preserving an established community. The cost of each project is returned to local government through the required repayment of rehabilitation loans.

"The elderly will no longer be herded into high-rise housing projects that encourage loneliness and introversion. Instead, their independence and outgoing spirit will be encouraged.

"Senior centers, with their wide range of services, will become even more integrated into the lives of the community's older people.

"Brandywine House is ideal for older persons who want their independence at reasonable cost. It may well be the forerunner of similar housing alternatives for the elderly in many other U.S. communities."

There are countless situations where people have discovered for themselves that two or more can live less expensively when resources are pooled. Congregate housing and communal living are examples of exciting and optimistic innovations for housing the nation's elderly.

Adult Day Care

Adult day care originated about 15 years ago as an offshoot of day care for mentally and emotionally impaired persons.

Elderly adults attend the day care center for part or all of the day. The program may be limited to crafts and social activities, with a hot meal in the middle of the day, or it may offer all-encompassing care of aged adults. Some centers offer breakfast, personal care (showers and shampoos for those who need this help), and even financial counseling. All of this is done to keep people out of nursing homes and functioning independently.

Day care centers are found in nursing homes, hospitals, and in separate buildings. The residents of nursing homes do not use a day care center even though it may be located in their facility. However, many people who use a nursing home center have a more comfortable transition to the nursing home when this move becomes necessary because they are familiar with the building and the staff.

Admission to a day care center must be approved by a physician.

In the next chapter you will find interviews with a director of an adult day care center and a day care supervisor who runs a program within a nursing home.

How Families React to Nursing Home Placement

Many families object to sending an aged relative away to a nursing home to receive professional care. Advising the family to do so requires skilled and supportive counseling.

If the symptoms of mental or physical impairment have become severe enough to create a serious problem, a protective environment is usually the only feasible answer. Many families who truly want their aged relative at home don't realize the enormous difference between their willingness to do this and their actual ability to carry out the task. The 24-hour care that is generally required can physically and emotionally exhaust the most loving caregivers.

Many old people with severe brain damage or physical problems that cannot easily be cared for at home can benefit from and even enjoy being in a nursing home because it: 1) is physically safe; 2) eliminates loneliness through increased social contact; and 3) has facilities for games, hobbies, and other activities that may stimulate their interest.

There are, of course, some geriatric patients who are bitter and unhappy no matter how ideal the conditions and skillful the care.

Families often have severe reactions when they've made the difficult decision to institutionalize an elderly relative. Some factors which influence these reactions are:

a low opinion of nursing homes

culture, ethnicity

disagreement within the family about what is best for the elderly relative

a feeling of having failed the elderly relative

a feeling of guilt when relief is experienced after institutionalization is achieved

Less frequent, but still significant, is the situation in which alternative living arrangements such as communal living, day care, or congregate housing have never been explored. The aged relative is simply "placed" in a nursing home when his or her circumstances or behavior become a problem.

Choosing a Nursing Home

Choosing a nursing home is a task that makes most people cringe. Yet, reality has to be faced. A group of practical nursing students was asked to pretend that a close family member needed a nursing home, and to indicate what criteria they would use in making a choice. The most important considerations to emerge from the group were cost, location, and staff attitudes.

Nearly every student could foresee financial problems and the need for assistance from social services. If the facility was easily accessible, family visits could be more frequent and of longer duration. The students felt that staff attitudes were significant for reasons that ranged from the philosophy of the administration to how well the nursing staff could recognize residents' potential. All the students saw a need for more than custodial care. Individuality and sexual identity (maintaining femininity and masculinity) through dress and grooming were considered important.

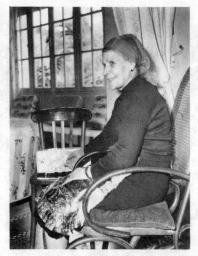

Woman who made a successful adjustment to living in a nursing home. She brought some personal belongings (a rocker, radio, and pillows) with her.   Courtesy of Skippy Gurau.

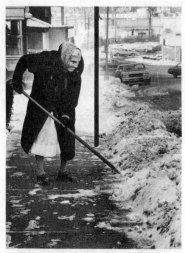

Eighty-nine year-old woman shovels snow in front of her home. Courtesy of Ed Malley.

Other significant student comments were concerned with:

Provisions for Privacy.   The resident doesn't have to have a private room, but there should be some place for his or her personal belongings. The trauma of relinquishing home and independence might be eased if a favorite chair or treasured keepsake stayed with the patient.

Making Preliminary Visits.   When looking for a nursing home for a relative, one should visit during all shifts and use all five senses. Check for odors that might mean poor hygienic practices. Touch counter tops, bedrails, and wheelchairs to be sure they are clean and not crusted with dried food and spilled liquids. Listen to staff talking to patients.

Dietary Considerations.   The habits and preferences of the patients should be taken into consideration whenever possible. Patients are confined and one of the few things they have to look forward to each day is mealtime. In fact, one student said that she would only choose a nursing home for her 86-year-old grandfather that would permit him to have his customary afternoon manhattan.

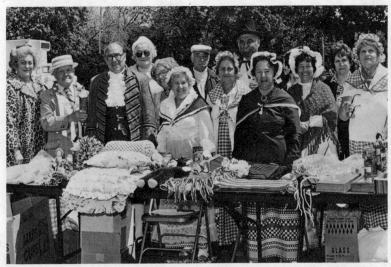

Staff and residents of a nursing home celebrating the country's bicentennial with a bazaar. Courtesy of Charles Carson.

Community Involvement. Some secondary schools participate in regular nursing home visits. Also, many nursing homes have gotten acquainted with the community through craft sales and bazaars. An opportunity to share a particular talent with the community can fulfill the need to feel useful—a need often denied to nursing home residents.

Spiritual Life. The religious needs of people must be met. In the later years, religion often assumes a new importance. Many nursing homes have rooms (or space in a room) set aside for religious services of different denominations.

The students also said that they would observe the staff to see if they took pride in their appearance and were neat and well groomed, the implication being that their appearance would be reflected in the care given to the residents.

Since the nurse is a resource person, she is sometimes asked how to choose a nursing home. The students' comments just listed will be helpful to the nurse when her advice is sought, as will the information listed below.

Start the Search

After discussing the needs of the person who requires the services of a nursing home with the physician, the best way to proceed is to list the facilities that seem suitable. Talk to friends, neighbors, the local medical society, the community welfare council, and to health and welfare departments. Even your church or temple is a reference point. When the initial groundwork is done, plan to visit those homes which seem to meet your requirements. Keep in mind, the home has to fit the patient, not the other way around!

Touring a Nursing Home

Look for:
1. a current state nursing home license
2. a current administrator's license
3. special services (hairdresser, barber, podiatrist, and so on)
4. financial assistance program

5. location
   a. near a hospital?
   b. convenient for family?
6. hazards
   a. lighting—is it adequate?
   b. safety rails—are they located in bathrooms and corridors?
   c. federal and state fire safety codes—are they enforced?
7. bedrooms
   a. are there four or fewer residents to a room?
   b. are call bells, fresh drinking water, reading lights by all beds?
   c. individual clothes closets and drawers?
8. cleanliness and lack of unpleasant odors
9. kitchens—are there separate areas for food preparation, dishwashing, and garbage disposal?
10. activity rooms?
11. examination rooms?
12. general atmosphere
    a. convenient visiting hours?
    b. does staff call patients by name?
13. Services
    a. is a physician available in an emergency?
    b. is physical therapy available?
    c. is a speech therapist available?
14. Activities (group and individual)
    a. do patients go on outside trips?
    b. are there volunteers in the home?

Financial Agreements

Be sure all financial agreements are in writing. There are several ways to meet financial requirements: social security payments, personal assets, welfare assistance, health insurance, and Medicare/Medicaid.

Types of Nursing Home Care

All legitimate nursing homes are licensed and regulated by the state in which they are located. State regulations vary greatly.

Nursing homes offer three types of service:
1. Nursing care utilizing the professional skills of nurses as well as physical therapy, diet therapy, and dental services.
2. Personal care, which means assistance with the activities of daily living.
3. Residential care, i.e., giving supervision for self-care residents. Level 4 homes (see box) are often called rest homes. To be eligible for acceptance into a rest home, the applicant must be well and must be able to take care of himself. Some rest homes are committed to life care of

---

Levels of Care: Basis for the Classification of Long Term Care Facilities

Level 1.   Intensive nursing and rehabilitative care facilities: these facilities provide skilled continuous care and an organized program of restorative services in addition to the minimum basic care and services.

Level 2.   Skilled nursing care facilities: these facilities provide continuous skilled nursing care and meaningful availability of restorative services and other therapeutic services in addition to the minimum basic care and services. They care for patients who show potential for improvement or restoration to a stabilized condition or who have a deteriorating condition that requires skilled care.

Level 3.   Supportive nursing care facilities: these facilities provide routine nursing services and periodic availability of skilled nursing, restorative, and other therapeutic services, in addition to the minimum basic care and services. They are for patients whose condition is stabilized to the point that they only need supportive nursing care, supervision, and observation.

Level 4.   Resident care facilities: these facilities provide protective supervision in addition to minimum basic care for residents who do not routinely require nursing or other medically related services.

---

residents. This means that if a resident becomes ill, he will be cared for in the home's infirmary, but there are no extraordinary measures—no IVs or respirators, for example. Infirmaries such as these give supportive care—even oxygen —but if more skilled nursing care is needed, the resident must go to a hospital.

All rest home residents are eligible for Medicare. Patients are all private-paying persons. Rest homes have sliding scales, however, and when social security and pensions don't cover the regular charges, adjustments are made by the home.

There are four levels of nursing home care (see box). Some homes offer only one level and others offer more than one.

Medicare/Medicaid

Medicare and Medicaid were legislated into existence in 1965. The differences between them are explained in the American Nursing Home Association's pamphlet, *Thinking About a Nursing Home?* as follows:

"Medicare, administered by the Social Security Administration, is a federal insurance program for persons 65 and over, persons disabled for at least two years, and persons suffering from chronic kidney diseases. Medicare will pay for nursing home care:

1. If the nursing home is certified as a Skilled Nursing Facility (SNF).
2. If the patient has spent at least three consecutive days in a hospital and provided the admittance to the SNF occurs within 14 days after discharge from the hospital.
3. If the physician certifies that extended care services are needed for the same or related illness for which the person was hospitalized; and
4. If continuous skilled nursing care or skilled rehabilitation services as defined by the Social Security Administration are required on a daily basis by the patient.

"If [all four of] the above requirements are met, the bill (for covered services only) can be paid by Medicare. Experts on

Medicare determine the amount to be paid, which the nursing home must accept in lieu of full payment, for the first 20 days in each benefit period. All but a small share per day can be paid for covered services for up to an additional 80 days if the patient qualifies.

"Each Medicare patient's case is under constant review by a committee of physicians as well as by the Social Security Administration. If these reviewers determine that the patient no longer requires professional nursing care and services, Medicare payments are ended.

"Medicaid, on the other hand, is a federal-state financed assistance program for certain needy and low income persons of all ages. States design their own Medicaid programs within broad federal guidelines. Medicaid programs will vary from state to state and individuals are encouraged to consult their own state or local welfare offices.

"If you need to find out who Medicare and/or Medicaid will cover and for how long, the most up-to-date resource personnel are in hospitals' social service departments. Other resource personnel can be found in your local health department, Council on Aging, Social Security Administration office, Visiting Nurse group, and Council of Churches."

The Rights of Patients

Human rights is a sensitive issue. Wars have been fought to defend dignity; people have died defending their integrity. In the 1960s, a decade marked by upheaval, rights again became a political cause. Who doesn't remember the savage scenes on campuses across the country of buildings seized and occupied and administrators barred from their offices?

Less dramatic but equally important are the day-to-day rights of patients in health care facilities. For many years, hospitals and physicians have had a paternalistic attitude toward patients, but this is changing. Acknowledging a patient's rights is an important part of the healing process.

Senior Citizen's Bill of Rights*

Each of our senior citizens, regardless of race, color, or creed, is entitled to:

The right to be useful.

The right to freedom from want in old age.

The right to obtain employment, based on merit.

The right to a fair share of the community's recreational, educational, and medical resources.

The right to obtain decent housing suited to the needs of later years.

The right to the moral and financial support of one's family so far as is consistent with the best interests of the family.

The right to live independently, as one chooses.

The right to live and die with dignity.

The right to access to all knowledge as available to improve the later years of life.

* *Prelude to A Senior Citizen's Bill of Rights, adopted at the 1961 White House Conference on Aging.*

What Is a Right?

By "right" we mean something enforceable in a court of law. Where there is a right there is a corresponding duty which can be legally enforced.

When a patient is admitted to a hospital or nursing home, he forfeits certain freedoms. For example, he loses the freedom of mobility because he may not wander in and out of hospital rooms or from floor to floor. A hospital gown is substituted for his own clothing. Unfortunately, sometimes a room number is even substituted for his name. (Have you ever heard a nurse say, "X-ray just called for 320B"?) Meals are served at the convenience of the hospital and even bedtimes seem to be scheduled. Obviously, there must be structure and regulation in patient care or chaos would result. However patients have the right to determine how they are to be treated.

In 1972, the Division of Nursing of the American Hospital

Association presented, for the first time anywhere, a Patients' Bill of Rights. The preamble states "These rights will be supported by the hospital on behalf of its patients as an integral part of the healing process. It is recognized that a personal relationship between the physician and the patient is essential for the provision of proper medical care." Patients' rights rest on these basic premises.

Guarding Privacy

There are still daily violations. For example, one of the rights listed in the Patients' Bill of Rights reads: "The patient has the right to every consideration of his privacy concerning his own medical care program. Case discussion . . . [is] confidential and should be conducted discreetly." Yet, Mrs. Y, a 65-year-old arthritic, was on her way to the X-ray Department in a large, modern medical center. She asked the young man wheeling her to stop at the nurses' station so she could ask for something for pain. Her physician was at the desk and overheard the request. He walked over to the patient and said, "Look, you have had enough medicine for the time being. I think you're making a mountain out of a molehill! You're not going to have anything more at this time." The patient was humiliated and even the orderly transporting the patient was embarrassed.

Another right reads: "The patient has a right to considerate and respectful care." However, in one 400-bed chronic care facility, patients who can stand are bathed standing naked at a sink in their rooms. Those awaiting tub baths are stripped naked and placed in a wheelchair, clutching a skimpy bath blanket to cover themselves. They wait in line in a drafty corridor until it is their turn to be bathed.

"The patient has a right to obtain from his physician complete and current information concerning his diagnosis, treatment and prognosis in terms he can be reasonably expected to understand." Yet, often a patient's query about his diagnosis and/or treatment is met with cliches such as, "Let *me* do the worrying," or, "It's nothing for you to be concerned with," or with medical jargon that completely bewilders people.

Righting the Wrongs

"Too little time," "not enough help" and "too many patients" have long been offered as excuses for the indignities and discomforts inflicted on patients. Since the Bill of Rights was first issued in 1972, hospitals and nursing homes all over the country have either adopted it or designed their own versions.

But there are still problems, and enforcement is difficult. Some states set fines for violations, but violations are not always easy to prove. Elsewhere, ombudsmen (officials empowered to investigate complaints about injustices or abuses) are the voices who speak for patients.

No document will ensure careful, considerate treatment for patients. Only people can do that. Health care professionals must work together to recognize the dignity of the individual.

Nursing Home Omburdsmen

In the early 1970s, the Department of Health, Education and Welfare introduced the concept of advocacy groups for nursing home residents. Each state has a Department of Elder Affairs and nursing home ombudsmen whose purpose is to investigate and resolve the complaints of nursing home residents.

This is where state uniformity ends, however. The state office may have ties on a municipal level with a Council of Churches, a Council on Aging, or a Home Care Corporation which, in turn, uses salaried or volunteer persons to fulfill advocacy goals.

What a Nursing Home Ombudsman Does

A nursing home ombudsman is a person who visits one or more nursing homes at least once a week for the purposes of getting to know the patients and staff, assessing the nursing home environment, and identifying problems in patient care. In talking to nursing home residents, the ombudsman is available to receive complaints. Problems are discussed with the nursing home administrator and/or the director of nursing. Problems that cannot be resolved by the nursing home staff are submitted to a coordinator of ombudsmen. Complaints received and the actions taken to resolve them are recorded on standardized forms.

Ombudsmen are given a training course during which some basic differences between nursing homes and hospital are stressed. One difference is that the nursing home resident has a much longer stay than a hospital patient with a resulting greater social isolation which causes a need for emotional attachment to persons other than staff and fellow residents.

Ombudsmen are counseled to keep relationships friendly but professional, and to respect the confidentiality of the patients and their diagnoses and treatments. They avoid criticism of the home, its personnel, and its policies, and they offer support and loyalty in a dignified, cordial, and businesslike manner.

Geriatric Care Abroad

A look at long term care in other countries can be useful to those of us interested in the aged. Europe has faced many of the same problems that affect geriatric care in this country. Lack of security in the big cities, the breakdown of the extended family, and economic instability are all factors that have influenced the rapid development of health care in the last few decades.

Great Britain, Denmark, and Sweden are countries that have implemented alternative noninstitutional living arrangements that have helped to solve many geriatric problems.

Before it instituted the National Health Service in 1949, England had a dismal record of caring for the elderly ill. They simply admitted old people to hospitals, kept them confined to beds, and, in most cases, didn't treat them. Eventually these people died either from the primary illness or from secondary problems.

Sweden had most of their elderly confined to poorhouses or nursing homes until the 1950s, when they developed alternative living arrangements for the aged. These include:

Loans to help modify an elderly person's home to accommodate his disabilities.

Housing allowances to permit elderly persons to select housing best suited to their needs.

Pensioner hotels, some with supervision.

Homes with continuous supervision and nursing service.

Denmark had a centuries' old tradition of taking care of their sick and aged relations at home. It was considered disgraceful to receive aid. That changed with various governmental policies in the early 1900s, and in the 1960s more sophisticated geriatric care was developed, for example, day care.

Two innovative European ideas are floating beds and rotating beds. Floating beds are beds that are held in a hospital for a limited period of time so that those who are caring for an elderly or infirm person can receive much-needed relief. Rotating beds are beds reserved in a hospital also. The family shares care with the hospital by having the patient at home for six weeks, then in the hospital for six weeks, then back in the home for another six weeks, and so on. When the system of rotating beds is used, efforts are extended to the family to encourage home care, i.e., certain remodeling (perhaps widening doorways to receive wheelchairs and installation of special plumbing) is paid for.

Many European countries recognize that geriatrics is a demanding speciality and, to attract competent and sufficient personnel in this discipline, a salary differential is offered.

DISCUSSION QUESTIONS

1. Many families experience severe guilt when they have made the decision to institutionalize an elderly relative. How can the nurse help the family deal constructively with this problem?
2. Mrs. X, 79, lived alone and independently until she fell at home and fractured her hip. She is now recovering from surgery in a hospital from which she will soon be discharged to a nursing home. Circumstances are such that nursing home placement will most likely be permanent.
    What physical and emotional problems can the nurse anticipate? What discharge planning can help ease the transfer from the hospital to the nursing home?

RESEARCH PROBLEM

1. As a clinical component of Chapter 2, select an elderly medical/-surgical patient to follow through discharge from the hospital. Research the discharge planning. Will your patient go home? Are support services needed? List and explain.
2. If your patient is going to a nursing home, why? What are the advantages? Disadvantages?
3. As a variation of this project, you might select a nursing home resident and investigate the circumstances that led to placement. Do you see alternatives? If so, why were they not used?

3

Personal Points of View

Objectives

After completing this chapter, the student should be able to:

- understand the circumstances under which people are admitted to nursing homes
- emphathize with the feelings of those who must place their parents in nursing homes
- begin to understand the problems of hospital social service workers who must direct recovered acute care patients to nursing homes
- appreciate the work done by adult day care centers

The material in this chapter gives a varied picture of the geriatric world. After reading each section, students should discuss it and evaluate the opinions it expresses.

Interview With a Nursing Home Administrator

"There are four main reasons why people are admitted to nursing homes: either the patient is living in an undesirable situation, which can mean he is living with a married son or daughter who doesn't want him, or he is living in a rundown apartment, or simply that he is unable to manage at home. *Or*, the patient is placed here by a son or daughter (maybe with great reluctance). Now the reaction from the person who comes from an undesirable situation is positive. This place [indicates his nursing home] looks like heaven after what he's been living with. But the patient who is *placed* here has a definite negative reaction. That patient feels he's been committed.

"We recognize that placement is difficult for both parents and children (and in some cases, spouses). We try to ease the transition from hospital or private home to nursing home as much as possible. The prospective resident is visited in the hospital by a social worker and a registered nurse. They objectively assess the elderly person. Then we have an orientation for patient and family. We also have monthly meetings with the families of our residents in groups; at these meetings we attempt to raise and examine any problems that the families may be facing.

"It's important to recognize that most families have great ambivalence about placement. They are almost invariably torn between feelings of relief and guilt when the placement is made.

"We have a supportive staff here. They realize that families as well as residents need encouragement. You know, the days are gone where a nurse was lowering herself to work in a nursing home. We consider geriatrics a dynamic specialty. Every once in a while we have a nurse or attendant leave because they are unsuited to this type of nursing. It's not dramatic work and our patients don't get better. Rarely is anyone discharged. The plain fact is that our patients *die*. Most of them die—unlike those in a hospital who recover and are discharged. Another problem we have from time to time is that our residents can lash out at an attendant racially or ethnically. Remember, these old people were living in an extremely prejudiced era. Of course, time will take care of this, but meanwhile the staff must be very patient. They have to realize what they're dealing with. They can't fight back! It takes a lot of patience."

The administrator was asked how he handled the situation of having a resident admitted to an acute care facility for care.

"This is a problem and about the only way to deal with it is the way our resident physician does. We get them into the hospital, have the problem taken care of, and get them back to the home as fast as possible. If we don't, we see confusion where there previously was no confusion. We see instant senility. It's very destructive. We have to face the fact that nursing home patients don't do well in hospitals if they have to stay there too long. I'll give you an example:

"Recently we had an 89-year-old resident admitted to the hospital because he had a blood clot in his leg. He nearly lost the leg. We were rather pessimistic. Well, in the course of his hospitalization he was seen by a surgeon, a medical man, a resident. He was visited by a dietitian, lab technicians, and x-ray technicians. Every shift brought a change of nurses! Finally, a young intern walked in and told the patient he was going to do a rectal. Well, the patient yelled, 'You idiot! It's not my ass, it's my leg!' He nearly went berserk. You see, he had had too much stimulation and not enough rest.

"We were all grateful to the hospital staff. After all, he got well; he didn't lose his leg!"

DISCUSSION QUESTIONS

1. Do you think the administrator is correct about the racial attitudes of some nursing home residents? How should nursing personnel react to racial abuse by residents?
2. Why does the administrator say that families are torn between feelings of relief and guilt when they place relatives in a nursing home?
3. What stereotypical social attitudes, other than racial attitudes, might a 70-, 80-, or 90-year-old nursing home resident hold?
4. Mr. B lives in a nursing home. He needs to be hospitalized for surgery. What are some problems to be anticipated when he is admitted? Suggest solutions.

Interview With a Woman Who Placed Her Father in a Nursing Home

"My father was one of 12 children and he came to this country from Austria when he was 14. He never went back. He prospered here, married and had two children—me and my brother. When we were very small, my grandmother was widowed and my father gladly took her into his home. I have memories of growing up with my grandmother always living with us.

"I had three young children when my mother died and my father came to live with us. At that time he was in his late 60s. He was with us for about two years when Parkinson's disease was diagnosed. Still, he was up and about and able to care for himself.

"Slowly he began to exhibit symptoms of senility. By that I mean he became confused, or he'd wander through the house during the night. Sometimes he'd stumble. He always would go to the children's room. Once he was there, he'd just stand and look at them. Often he'd touch them lightly on the cheek and sometimes he'd lean over and kiss them. Now this frightened the children. We knew he loved them, but they couldn't understand. Oh, we'd try to intercept him, but we didn't always hear him. Well, tensions arose and anxiety was transmitted from one to the other. We found ourselves becoming tense and irritable. My husband and I were always expecting him to fall over something and the children were developing erratic sleep patterns. They were awakening frequently during the night even when he didn't go in their room. Oh, there were other 'eccentric' behaviors, but the wandering and the effect on my children were unbearable.

"It was with a real heavy heart that I took him to a nursing home. I was tormented because I experienced the emotions of relief and guilt. Relief because we could now lead a normal family life and I didn't have to worry about father wandering away from the house or falling and hurting himself. Yet guilt because I was the first one in the family ever to put someone in a *home.* In my father's generation this was considered a disgrace. The last place anyone ever wanted to end up in was a home. My father had opened his home up to an aging parent and I turned out my own father!

"I rationalized, or you could say I absolved my guilt, by going daily to the nursing home. I'd bathe him, feed him breakfast, dress him, and later in the day I'd feed him lunch. Then I'd go home and care for my own family. My brother would come each evening and feed him dinner and then prepare him for the night.

"Now you know something strange? The reaction of the other residents of the home was one I wasn't prepared for. They were *jealous*! They'd always ask me, 'Why do you come every day? He isn't sick. You don't have to come every day. You're foolish to be babying him.' Remarks like that. Well, it was true that he wasn't in the throes of a last illness, but he did need care—the care I was unable to give him at home. More important, I needed a way to get rid of my own guilt. But they wouldn't have understood that.

"I noticed other things, too. Occasionally the staff would talk over him or about him *in his presence* and he would quite literally droop. He had some speech problems and he couldn't respond immediately to their questions or conversations. I found that just waiting patiently would allow enough time for the replies, but they were busy and rushed, so they didn't wait. They labeled him 'unable to respond'!

"If I were asked to give a word of advice to those who work in nursing homes (and I admit, it does take a special dedication) it would be to *listen* to the residents. Be patient and give them a chance to respond.

"Also, acknowledge whoever you see even if it isn't the person you came to visit. This is their *home.* A smile, a word of greeting, just a touch on the arm can mean so much to a resident who may rarely or may never have a visitor. Don't just pass them by as if they weren't even there. I know people don't mean to do this, and I understand, but I think visitors *and* staff have to consciously remind themselves to recognize the residents. To acknowledge them.

"My father has been dead for many years now, but I still have guilt. Why? Well, I'll tell you. He had a poor swallowing reflex, as do many patients with Parkinson's. One day he was fed by someone who didn't know how to feed him . . . and he choked."

DISCUSSION QUESTIONS

1. Why do you think the other patients were jealous of the attention this woman gave to her father?
2. Do you think most facilities would welcome a patient's relative doing as much for a patient as this woman and her brother did?
3. How can nursing homes encourage relatives to care for their invalids in nursing homes? Do you think relatives believe that the nursing homes wouldn't like them to do this?
4. What would be the proper procedure for feeding a patient who had a poor swallowing reflex?
5. When a rational patient has a speech problem and can't respond to a nurse immediately, what should the nurse do?

Interview With a Woman Who Placed Her Mother First in a Rest Home and Then in a Nursing Home

This interesting story is about a woman with arteriosclerosis and how her disease progressed from occasional forgetfulness to dangerously inappropriate behavior. Reading this should provide insight into some of the stress, frustration, and anxiety endured by family members as they observe the inevitable deterioration of an aged parent.

"To look at my mother you couldn't imagine a thing wrong with her. Outwardly she was a beautiful woman. But she had arteriosclerosis from the time she was just 62 years of age. I guess you could say it killed off her brain cells. She became forgetful. Very forgetful. As long as my father was alive he used to cover up for her, so we didn't notice it too much. At least not to the point where we did anything but joke about it.

"I used to bring all my clothes to her to be altered. One day I saw that she had unaccountably sheared off about three inches from a very expensive dress. That was my first indication that there was something really wrong with my mother. It was horrendous, both for me and for my father. You see, there was a 15-year age difference between them and my father always hovered over mother. When she became "ill," he took care of her like you would a retarded child . . . with tenderness, love, and protection. But then he died very suddenly. So, what was to become of mother? They had lived together for over 40 years in the home we were raised in. A big 12-room house. That house was their 'roots' and it seemed cruel to change things. But my brother and I had to face the fact that there was a serious problem. At this time we were both against the idea of a nursing home. In fact, it was unthinkable. We were busy enough selling the home and all the furnishings and accumulation of 40 years.

"Well, I decided that I could take care of her. I was working at the time but I decided to cut down to four days a week. I would take mother from Thursday to Monday and then my brother and his wife would take over the rest of the time.

"My sister-in-law had a job, too, and one day she came home to find that mother had taken all the drapes down and had hidden them. Then she'd forget that she'd eaten and would go to the refrigerator and eat enormous quantities. She'd eat seven meals a day and slowly she got enormously heavy. She was always accusing them of not giving her anything to eat.

"Another time she hid my husband's wallet. We had a terrible time trying to find it. Then she had a temper tantrum when I suggested she wear a hat to some function we had to attend. She actually threw the hat out of the window. All this was thoroughly uncharacteristic behavior for my mother. After all, my mother had been an impeccably dressed woman—every hair in place, weekly manicures. My mother never had a crooked seam or anything less than immaculately white gloves. Now it didn't bother her to wear the same dress five days in a row—food stains, ripped hems, torn stockings. It was very upsetting to all of us. It became such an emotional issue that we were forced to consider alternatives. We decided she wasn't bad enough for a regular nursing home, so we put her in a rest home. It was a mistake, but we didn't realize that until later.

"The home looked cozy enough and Mother had a nice room with a radio, TV, and attractive furnishings. But she'd wear the same dress every day until I came to change it. Of course I'd go four or five times a week to do her laundry, change her clothing, and kind of supervise. But it wasn't working out. There were 12 women residents and one attendant. It was perfectly fine for people who had their wits about them (they had room and board) but for my mother, well, she needed closer watching. If I didn't give her a bath she wouldn't have one. If I didn't dress her she'd wear the same thing all the time. Things came to a head when one day I took her shopping and got the shock of my life when she undressed. Her slip was dirty and everything she had on seemed to be soiled. It was embarrassing.

"Now you probably are wondering why we didn't do something right away. Well, when it's your mother, you come to those decisions slowly. At last my brother and I had her transferred to a place where she would be supervised in all her activities. The day she was to be transferred was a nightmare. She put up incredible resistance! She was like a woman possessed. She ranted and raved, she wouldn't get out of her easy chair (she was now massively obese). They just couldn't move her. She claimed that these people were trying to evict her from her own home and she refused to cooperate with any of us. She started to scream that she meant to stay here because my father was coming for her. We couldn't convince her that Dad was dead. She was totally out of control. My gentle mother, who never in her life said anything stronger than 'hell's bells,'' was spewing obscenities like we couldn't believe!

"When she became hysterical they trussed her up in what seemed to be some sort of straitjacket. Then they secured her to her chair and . . . I know you'll find this hard to believe, but it's true . . . they backed up a small pickup truck to the rest home, lifted her, chair and all, onto the truck, and transported her to the nursing home. In retrospect, it might have even looked funny to a passerby. Here's this old lady with beautiful snowy white hair tied in a chair in the back of a truck. They hauled her to her room and just placed her there. After a couple of hours she became quite subdued. I don't know why they didn't medicate her, but they didn't. I sat with her for the whole time and at last she looked at me and said, with tears in her eyes, 'Look what they did to me.' I can still hear her.

"The nursing home was spotless and the attendants were very good to her. But I want to warn *anyone* who has to put someone in a nursing home: don't think for a minute that just because the home is expensive, clean, and attractive that you can just forget to visit and visit frequently! I was there four or five times a week, not only to see my mother but to indicate by my being there that I expected care to be given, that I expected them to do what we were paying for (and it took every last cent we had!).

"Now I'll tell you the problems. One day I noticed that my mother was having trouble walking. She couldn't tell me what was wrong; she could only grimace and limp and I figured it out for myself. I took off her shoes and stockings and I nearly died. Her toenails hadn't been cut in nearly a year. They had grown *under* her toes. Now, I was shocked and disappointed because I expected that at some time a nurse or *someone* would have looked at her feet. We got a podiatrist right away and made arrangements for a monthly visit with him.

"There was another unhappy situation in which a black nurse wanted my mother to get undressed for a shower. My mother, in her state of confusion, interpreted this as a sexual attack and became enraged. She had had blacks as servants and never thought of them as equals; therefore, in anger and in ignorance, she began name calling and lashing out at the nurse. While people were trying to restrain her, her glasses were broken, she fell and received bruises—oh, it was a mess.

"I had a bad experience with the physician in charge. Apparently the tranquilizer she was on didn't affect her. The doctor said he was making arrangements to commit her to the state mental hospital. I was furious. He said he didn't want to be bothered with her aggressiveness. Well, I said, 'That's your problem. She has a debilitating, degenerative disease and she'll die from it. We know that and we've accepted it. But if you don't try to help her by at least trying another medication, I'll go to my senator, my congressman, the newspapers, everybody!'

"The final incident happened about a month after. I noticed that mother felt quite warm and was listless. I called it to the attention of the nurse and she said that they were watching her. I called the doctor (by now he had me labeled as a troublemaker) and he just said, 'Don't worry about it; let me worry about it.' I went home upset and, don't you know, about 11 PM that night I received a call that mother had been admitted to the hospital with pneumonia. She died a few days later.

"If I could make one point I would say *become involved.* Don't just tuck a person away and forget about him. Ask questions. Don't be brushed off. And above all, be there. See what's happening. They'll respect you for it and you'll know you did the right thing."

DISCUSSION QUESTIONS

1. Do you think that this woman's mother's doctor was typical in viewing her as a troublemaker?   Do you think he was right or wrong?
2. How can you account for the rest home keeping this woman when she was obviously so confused?
3. Do you think this woman could, at times, appreciate what her daughter was doing for her?

Interview With a Hospital Social Service Director

"One of the most difficult things we have to do is get the patient to accept the fact that he can't go home. That he *needs* a nursing home. After all, it's hard to admit you can't go home and manage. We have to get right down to basics and, for example, we ask, 'Can you walk to the bathroom?' 'Can you prepare a meal?' Even, 'Can you get out of bed?'

"Just to make sure we know what we're dealing with, we have to go to the patient's room and ask the nurse to show us exactly what the patient can do. And we watch closely.

"Home care can be very expensive and it's not always practical. The most home care that people on welfare can expect is about eight hours a day. Usually they get four hours. That leaves them alone to manage the best they can the rest of the day. Now, unless they're pretty independent, or there is family around, that small block of time with a homemaker isn't very much help. It really doesn't do much good.

"On the other hand, if they can get around and they just need someone to do housework and get meals, then they can manage with four hours a day. Someone will come in, get them ready for the day, do a little light housework, fix a hot meal, and leave something in the refrigerator for supper. That type of situation works out.

"But acceptance is the hardest part. We usually tell them that going to a nursing home is a temporary arrangement because many times it is. We don't want anyone to feel they're going someplace forever. We tell them that they will get more therapy (as in the case of a patient with a stroke or a fractured hip) in the nursing home, and that the goal is to continue the care that they got in the hospital (emphasizing the therapy) until they are more independent and then they can get along, although at a slower pace.

"In an acute care hospital they have to have acute care. When they reach a point where they don't need this kind of care, then they can be taken care of just as well someplace else. Medicare provides Level One nursing home care for this kind of (acute) patient. If the patient doesn't need this kind of care, then maybe a Level Three category (supportive nursing care) is all that's needed. That is a different situation.

"When Medicare first went into effect, a patient had 100 days coverage in an extended care facility. Then, if you were in a hospital for three days, or you required a nursing home for care following hospitalization, you could get transferred to a Level One nursing home. You were allowed to stay there for 100 days and you got 100 days coverage. Today the rules are so stringent that there are very few people who qualify for Level One Medicare coverage in a nursing home. The patient must require skilled care, and the interpretation of skilled care is strict. For example, a fractured hip patient in a hospital who is ambulatory with a walker will not be covered for *any* care at all. But if he needs physical therapy in order to learn to walk with the walker, then he will be covered for therapy in a Level One home until he improves. But watch out! If he reaches a plateau, the benefits can be stopped. If patients go two or three weeks and don't improve, Medicare will not pay for skilled care at that point.

"Another example: if a patient needs oxygen, he must require oxygen *around the clock.* It can't be oxygen as needed. If he needs injections, it has to be every four hours. Dressings that have to be changed regularly will be covered in a Level One nursing home.

"Rehabilitation seems to be the key for Level One coverage. But not all rehabilitation is covered. For example, if you had a stroke patient who subsequently fell and fractured his hip, that patient probably would not be considered rehabilitative and therefore would not be covered.

"Cost is the deciding factor in most Level One nursing homes. These nursing homes will take private patients ahead of welfare patients. It's very difficult to get welfare patients in ahead of private patients because reimbursement is poor.

"Families are ambivalent about putting an elderly parent in a nursing home. We try to point out that there comes a time when you just can't manage. It would be doing a disservice to the family to keep the patient at home. We've seen situations where people neglect their own spouses or children in order to care for an elderly parent, and we try to give them support in making the difficult decision of placing the parent in a nursing home. Frequently, people who are caring for aged parents reach the point where they can no longer handle the person physically and then they make the decision for placement.

"Oh, we have seen all kinds of situations. Patients can refuse to go to families who want them. Families can refuse to care for patients they really could manage. We've heard all kinds of stories. But we aren't judgmental because we don't always know the situation at home. I have a case right now where a young mother is considering placement for her aged father. She's come to see me several times to discuss this and each time I see her she has a new excuse why she can't keep her father at home. The stairs, the noise of the children (she has three little boys), and so on and so on. Finally, I had to say to her, "Look, this is your decision. You don't have to explain to me if you really don't feel you can handle this. Your own family is probably too much responsibility for you right now." There aren't many people who don't have heavy guilt feelings about placing a parent in a nursing home. We have to reassure them that keeping the patient home isn't always the answer. Maybe the patient wouldn't be getting the proper care, therapy, and so on, if they took him home. After all, it's a 24-hour responsibility. It can wreck a family, and there are things that a nursing home can do that the family can't.

"For a long time we saw a trend where elderly patients almost routinely went to nursing homes from the hospital. Now we see that changing. We find that more patients are going home with some type of home care. Our philosophy here is to send everybody home we can. We want to maintain people at home because usually they're going to do their best at home. However, if it doesn't work out, we look for alternatives."

DISCUSSION QUESTIONS

1. Compare the nursing home administrator's comment (page 40) that "The plain fact is that most of our patients die,'' with the social service director's remark (page 49) that "We usually tell them that going to a nursing home is a temporary arrangement because many times it is." Who do you think is more accurate? Why would their points of view be so different?
2. Why do you suppose so many people feel guilty about placing an elderly relative in a nursing home whereas they wouldn't feel guilty about placing him in a hospital?

Interview With a Geriatric Nurse

"This is a private-pay, Level Two and Three nursing home. At a glance, you would have to say it looks great here—the decor, the lounges for the residents, the activities available. Our dietitian sees all the residents daily and tries very hard to accommodate everybody.

"I've been working here seven years and I truly love it. I work hard, but there is not the pressure of hospitals. We do have some problems, however. For one, we have no full-time nurses. Oh, I tried it, but I just couldn't keep it up. We have no orderly, so we are responsible for all our lifting and moving. I have wonderful nurses to work with, but we have a problem with our assistants.

The aides. We hire them right off the streets. Now, that means that for every ten you train (on-the-job training), you have maybe one that stays with you. The others, well, some we have to let go. They aren't rude to the residents, but they just have no feeling for this type of work. Others have an extremely high absentee rate.

"To get back to the nurses; the reason we have no full timers is that everyone feels as I do. The sameness of geriatrics becomes a pressure when you don't have enough help. Pay definitely has to be upgraded here. If we could attract a better quality, *trained* aide, that would make a tremendous difference. I think education is the only way to solve the problem of geriatric nursing today. Here we feel that the hospital RN or LPN looks down on those of us who prefer working in a nursing home. I've heard it said that many think we couldn't get work anywhere else. Well, that's not true. Every nurse here, to the best of my knowledge, is here because she loves geriatric patients. We take time to listen to our residents. It becomes frustrating, though, when you find yourself working shorthanded. When that happens I always say to the residents, "I'll be back," and I make every effort to get back to them. But it can bother you. All of the residents have their own needs. Some are lonesome, some are depressed. You can't just hand out a pill and forget about them.

"We don't have the dramatic recoveries here that take place in hospitals. But we do see changes that make this work very rewarding. We have a woman here who came in to us a year ago bedridden and unresponsive. She was like a vegetable. We got her as a transfer from another nursing home. Well, it turned out that at one time she had had seizures so she was put on Dilantin. They examined her Dilantin levels and found that they were excessive. After she was off the Dilantin she slowly showed improvement until now she can walk a few steps with assistance and she is lucid. She had been practically comatose. We have another resident, a gentleman who came to us with a Foley catheter and a nasogastric tube in place. In less than six months he was continent and eating well.

"I'm 55 and I will never leave here. But the only way I see the future of geriatric nursing improving is to attract younger nurses. The only way that will be done is if students have more emphasis on geriatrics in their education. It is *not* second-rate nursing. It's challenging, a fertile field for innovative techniques, and extremely satisfying. The future of geriatrics lies in the nursing schools.''

DISCUSSION QUESTION

1.   Suggest ways to motivate nurses to enter the field of geriatric nursing.

Interview With a Former Inspector of Nursing Homes

The inspector gives a cynical but, he claims, realistic view of the nursing home situation.

"I was hired by the state to visit homes and examine them for physical requirements—fire exits, temperature of the water, bed brakes, and other safety features. I was also to observe nursing care. Well, as you can imagine, that's hard to do because you *always* seem to be filling out forms. I used to ask my supervisor to let me forget the forms and just go in and work in the home a few days, throw back the covers, that sort of thing. *Then* I would feel that I could give an accurate evaluation. But we don't do that. There isn't enough time.

"The nusing homes don't know exactly when we will inspect them, but if their license is ready to expire in October, they start getting ready in August—with their records, that is. The emphasis is always on paperwork.

"I warn you in advance—I went into inspection with ideals and high hopes. I've emerged sadder and wiser. Let me tell you what I found disillusioning.

"While there are good nursing homes with caring staffs, I found too many situations where the business came first and the residents a poor second. I found a rest home where the residents had to buy their own toilet paper. Where they had to pay 15 cents to make a 10-cent phone call! (I came on this accidentally because I was sitting at a small desk, filling out a form, when a resident shuffled up to me, handed me 15 cents while he used the phone. When I asked him what was happening, he told me that everybody was required by the administrator to pay 15 cents for a call). At this same rest home, I checked the kitchen and observed the chef preparing two pounds of liver for 16 people! When I expressed surprise and dismay, he nervously agreed to prepare other meat that (together) we found in the refrigerator. Clearly, he was afraid of repercussions. On another occasion I was informed that a slightly retarded resident was forced to do housework there.

"As you can imagine, I was determined to change things. I wrote memos, I even refused to relicense them. I sent a letter of violation. This last requires that the nursing home respond to the deficiencies. My supervisor was aghast because in the event that the home doesn't respond, then there is a hearing and the nursing home attends with legal counsel. The inspector, however, goes alone! I was advised never to get involved in a hearing because the lawyers can make the inspectors look foolish.

"Nothing ever happened. My memos went unanswered, the home never responded to the letter of violation, and the hearing was postponed many months until the home simply went out of business. They never improved conditions, they just transferred the 16 people and closed their doors.

"At another nursing home, I found a blatant violation in which the food and laundry areas were not separated; laundry was all over the floor in the kitchen where the washer and dryer were kept. Again, memos, reports, and so on, and nothing was done.

"I went to visit a large, municipal facility for the indigent aged and purely by chance I was present at an incident I will never be able to forget. It was lunch time and the nurses and attendants were feeding patients. I walked by one room where an attendant was literally shoveling food into a confused, restrained patient who was coughing and spitting. As I stood there watching, she slapped the man! I was rigid with shock and anger and I cried, 'What do you think you are doing?' With this, the aide turned to me and said, 'He's a force feed . . . he must eat.' I notified the supervisor and the director of nurses. I wrote a report that accurately described the incident and I was told that disciplinary measures would be taken. I assumed the woman would be fired, but I was wrong. She was just suspended for a few days. A year later, when I checked that facility again, to my amazement the same aide was there. I hurried down to the administrator and went over the whole story. He then proceeded to tell me that the attendant, who had recently emigrated to the United States, had had a language barrier at the time and he felt that changed the circumstances. They had agreed to soft-pedal the incident, he said, because in her culture people treated each other quite 'roughly,' was the way he put it. But he assured me that she was being closely watched and any other misstep would cause her immediate dismissal. For all I know, she's still there.

"The picture isn't bleak, but it bears watching. Many nursing homes sincerely try but they're handicapped financially. They have a difficult time getting the help they need and *want*. I know a nursing home administrator who is a very caring person. Been in the field for several years and has done a lot of good. Now he's thinking of leaving because he's so hampered by regulations and lack of funds."

When the young man was questioned as to the place of ombudsmen in nursing homes he replied:

"I know what you mean. The volunteer visitor ombudsman attempts to respond to patients' concerns and see that their needs are being met. And I have heard of cases where they have investigated and resolved complaints made by elderly individuals or made by persons concerned with a particular situation in a long term care facility. I've been told that they try to find legal resources for specific problems that can't be resolved or answered easily without legal assistance. Personally, I feel that there is a need for them *but* my gut feeling (and it probably stems from my three frustrating years as an inspector) is that patients and families are reluctant to talk to them. I feel that there is always the threat of retaliation hanging over their heads. You know — 'If I tell the ombudsman, then they'll take it out on my mother or wife.' This is what I honestly feel."

When asked what could be done, what measures might be taken to tighten the inspection procedure and the policies on violation, he responded:

"I'm pessimistic. These jobs with the state are good jobs. They pay well, you have nice hours, freedom in which to pursue your responsibilities (in terms of which nursing home I will visit when), benefits, you are building a pension, and so on. You look at your superiors and you say, 'I could be there if I don't rock the boat.' So the state encourages a philosophy of keeping the status quo. And don't forget, when you work for the state, there are always political influences to take into consideration."

DISCUSSION QUESTIONS

1. If you were aware of a serious nursing home violation in a place where you worked, what would you do? If you were a patient's relative and were aware of such a violation, what would you do?

2. Do you think the inspector is right when he says that ombudsmen can't be effective because patients and their families are afraid of retaliation? If so, how can this be changed?

Interview With a Director of an Adult Day Care Center

"This center is just like a nursing home except that our clients go home at 4 PM. When they come in in the morning (a van brings them to the center) they have juice, coffee, and toast. We also offer complete grooming services if they need it. We have a shower room and attendants who assist with showers, hair care, and oral hygiene if necessary. We serve a hot meal at noon, also. We offer all kinds of crafts along with day trips, and even weekend trips in some instances. We encourage, but don't force, involvement.

"We get our referrals from VNA, Homemakers, and physicians. I guess our only restrictions are incontinency and confusion that would be disturbing to others. We aren't equipped to handle either of those situations. I'm not saying that we don't have anyone who isn't confused—we do. But it is not disruptive.

"People seek this center for several reasons. We have many here who need to socialize. They live alone and it is good for them to be with other people. We have some who are retarded. There is one elderly woman who lives with her younger sister. Day care gives the sister some relief. We have another younger woman who lives alone. She has a family but they aren't interested in her. We offer many services to this client. Grooming, as I mentioned, and we even help her with her laundry. [A washer and dryer are installed in the center for those who need to use these appliances.] We have had to supervise her budgeting of her social security money because we discovered that she was being taken advantage of. You see, she bought a stereo on time and it so happened that she was *over*paying on her installments. Currently we are also teaching her to diet. She's anxious to lose weight, so diet teaching is another need to be filled.

"When we get referrals, we do individual interviews in the homes. I know of very few cases where the reaction to our center has been negative. Alcoholism sometimes presents a problem. Don't misunderstand me—alcoholism isn't a deterrant to coming here. We have several alcoholics but they cause no disturbance to our other clients. The problem we experienced with some alcoholics, however, was that of missing time here. They would be accepted, then miss a day, then more days, and finally not show up at all.

"Most of our experiences have been rewarding. There is a need here for day care and it's going to increase because the population of elderly is increasing. We are now accommodating all we can and we see a need for another day care center."

DISCUSSION QUESTIONS

1. If you were elderly and lived alone, do you think you would enjoy going to a day care center? Why or why not?
2. If you were to visit an adult day care center, what do you think it would be like?
3. Do you think the term "day care center" implies that the people who go to these centers are childish? If so, do you think that some elderly people might resent that name? Can you think of a better one?

Interview With a Day Care Supervisor
Who Runs a Program Within a Nursing Home

"Day care is an alternative to a nursing home. Sometimes people are in nursing homes inappropriately. It happens this way: at one time an acute condition required nursing home placement, but now perhaps it is a chronic condition that actually could be taken care of at home. The trend today is to take people out of the nursing home if they were inappropriately placed there.

"Day care may be used as a transition. Some go from the nursing home to day care and then to their own home. Day care is also useful for people who come from a hospital situation (say, after having had a stroke)because they can have all their therapies here. We have physical therapy, speech therapy, diet therapy and, most important of all, we have good peer socialization.

"We find that many elderly people are very depressed. In fact, we have had some that were suicidal. For whatever reason, they simply cannot cope with their disabilities or infirmities. We have excellent social services in this facility and that, plus peer socialization, is therapeutic in relieving depression.

"Another purpose for day care is family relief. Caring for a confused, forgetful person 24 hours a day is too much. The family needs relief.

"Sometimes when families come into the home asking for an application for the nursing home, it isn't appropriate. Not at that time. Maybe day care can answer the need until such time as when they have to go into a nursing home.

"In order to be accepted into day care, patients must be approved by a physician. This is a medically approved program. Then, if they are medically approved, they may also have to be approved by the Medicaid office. (Most of these participants are Medicaid patients.) It just isn't enough to say they are lonely and need other people around them. It's not a drop-in center; we have a structured program, you see. People come for reasons of their infirmities or disabilities or advanced depression. Not just because they are a little lonely.

"Most of these people, while they live independently on the outside, can't just pick up and go downtown on a bus. Sometimes it's because of finances. Some can't afford a phone. And, basically, they need their own peer group around them. They need to be involved in things in order to prove their own worth. People this age feel they aren't worth anything anymore. They feel that they are just a burden to their families. But here they become involved.

"They aren't doing fingerpainting, either! We accomplish meaningful activities. We teach the activities of daily living, how to make a bed and cook if you're handicapped. And we also involve them in some things they've never done before. We have art classes, we go bowling and even swimming. For many of our people, it's a first.

"The concept of day care began in Baltimore about 15 years ago. It started with mental patients who were taken during the day (if the families worked during the day) or at night, if the families couldn't keep them home at night.

"This age group we have here—60 to 90—still feels that a nursing home is a place where you go to die. It's a last resort. Yet, we have had people living in our nursing home 15, 16 years! This is not just custodial care. They are living.

"We are always arranging to go out. We go to plays, to picnics, out to dinner, other functions. And we have all kinds of volunteers. We have people come in to do makeup, manicures, help them shop for clothes. Half of our people live by themselves, and the other half live with their children or spouses.

"We have also found marriages that were very unstable. They were the kind of marriage that managed until something went wrong (like poor health) and then got very shaky. Sometimes we had to intervene through social services.

"Day care got off to a slow start here in New England about six years ago but within a few years centers sprouted up all over and they are all booked. They all have waiting lists.

"We have also had people who reacted negatively to day care. Perhaps they couldn't accept structure or maybe they wanted *more* structure. There were others who wanted to come and go as they pleased. For some the day was too long.

"I find that now we are taking on a much sicker clientele. We had one lady last year who had four heart attacks before she had her fifth one right here. It wasn't as upsetting as you might think. Oh, we did feel sad but, remember, this is a group who is very realistic about death. One man said, "Well, Edna always said her biggest fear was that she would die alone. And look! She died among all her friends.'

"Any nursing home that wished to develop a day care center would have to contact the Department of Public Welfare. They in turn send criteria which has to be satisfied before anything further can be done. Then you are either approved or not approved.

"A rate-setting commission sets fees. People who qualify for

Medicaid are completely paid for by the state. Their program and their transportation are both paid. But they must meet the criteria of being Medicaid approved. The others are private paying. Some are on fixed incomes that are just slightly above what the state allows for Medicaid and I have a problem with that. It costs $13 a day for the program and $3 for transportation. I feel we are almost taking food out of their mouths. Some really can't afford this and they go without to come here. I'm always trying to get 'scholarships' for them. I would definitely prefer a sliding fee. I think it would be fairer. But, so far, nothing.

"Now, for people who hold private insurance policies with an insurance company or Blue Cross Extended Care, 80 percent is paid for. We are getting more people interested in and paying for day care.

"Our aim for day care here is to get the patients to function independently. We want them to live on the outside for as long as possible. We have discharged people from this program, people who are better. For example, we had a man here not too long ago who had a stroke and a pelvic fracture. He came here, had all his therapies here, and we discharged him back into the community. I brought him to the community center for swimming and to the drop-in center so he could get his meals. He is now driving and he comes to us as a volunteer twice a week. We don't lose anyone. They all come back. We had another man in a deep depression after he lost his wife. Then he fell and fractured his hip. He came back here, had all his therapies, and, best of all, we worked through the grieving process with him. He volunteers here five days a week in woodworking. He teaches it to our people here in the program.

"An innovation in day care, as I mentioned before, is to get the patient out of the nursing home and back into the community. This is a comfortable transition. It also works the other way around. When a person who is coming to day care reaches the point when nursing home admission is necessary, the move into our nursing home is not as traumatic. For one thing, a new admission already knows most of our staff and, best of all, there are friends here. My day care group knows many, many residents. I guess you could say we bridge the gap between dependence and independence in more ways than one."

Note: Day care directors get together formally and informally many times during the year. They share ideas and review innovations, goals, and philosophies. As one day care supervisor said, "The hospital takes care of one problem but we take care of the total person."

DISCUSSION QUESTION

1.   Name all the reasons you can think of why day care would be good for elderly patients who do not belong in hospitals or nursing homes.

Letter From a Nursing Home Resident

Hello! Is there anyone out there who will listen to me? How can I convince you that I am a prisoner? For the past five years I have not seen a park or the ocean or even just a few feet of grass.

I am an 84-year-old woman and the only crime I have committed is that I have an illness which is called chronic. I have severe arthritis and five years ago I broke my hip. While I was recuperating in the hospital I realized that I would need extra help at home. But there was no one. My son died 35 years ago and my husband 25 years ago. I have a few nieces and nephews who come by to visit once in a while, but I couldn't ask them to take me in, and the few friends I still have are just getting by. So I wound up in a convalescent hospital in Los Angeles.

All kinds of people are thrown together here. I sit and watch, day after day. As I look around this room, I see the pathetic ones (maybe the lucky ones) who have lost their minds and the poor souls who should be out but nobody comes to get them, and the sick ones who are in pain. We are all locked up together.

I have been keeping in touch with the world through the newspaper, my one great luxury. For the last few years I have been reading about the changes in Medicare regulations. All I can see from these improvements is that nurses spend more time writing. For, after all, how do you regulate caring?

Most of the nurses' aides who work here are from other countries. Even those who can speak English don't have much in common with us. So, they hurry to get their work done as quickly as possible. There are a few caring people who work here, but there are so many of us who are needy for that kind of honest attention.

A doctor comes to see me once a month. He spends three to five seconds with me and then a few more minutes writing in the chart or joking with the nurses . . . I sometimes wonder how the aides feel when they work so hard for so little money and then see that the one who spends so little time is the one who is paid the most.

. . . most of the physicians who come here don't even pay attention to things like whether their patients' fingernails are trimmed or whether their body is foul smelling . . . . I hadn't had a bath in ten days . . . the aide wrote in the chart that she gave me a shower. Who would check or care? I would be labeled as a complainer or as losing my memory, and that would be worse.

As I write this, I keep wishing I were exaggerating. These last five years feel like the last five hundred of my life . . . . How can I tell you that for me growing old in America is an unbelievable, lonely nightmare?

I am writing this because many of you may live to be old like me, and then it will be too late. You too will be stuck here and wonder why nothing is being done, and you too will wonder if there is any justice in life.

Right now I pray every night that I may die in my sleep and get this nightmare of what someone has called life over with if it means living in this prison day after day.

—Anonymous letter to the *Los Angeles Times,* October, 1979

What Do You See, Nurses? *

What do you see, nurses? What do you see?
What are you thinking when you're looking at me?
A crabbit old woman, not very wise,
Uncertain of habit, with faraway eyes.
Who dribbles her food, and makes no reply
When *you* say in a loud voice, "I do wish you'd try."
Who seems not to notice the things that you do,
And forever is losing a stocking or shoe.
Who, unresisting or not, lets you do as you will

When bathing and feeding—the long day to fill.
Is that what you're thinking? Is that what you see?
Then open your eyes, nurse, you're not looking at *me*.
I'll tell you who I am as I sit here so still;
As I drink at your bidding and eat at your will.
I'm a small child of ten, with a father and mother,
Brothers and sisters who love one another.
A young girl of sixteen, with wings on her feet,
Dreaming that soon, now, a lover she'll meet.
A bride at twenty; my heart gives a leap,
Remembering the vows I promised to keep.
At twenty-five now, I have young of my own,
Who need me to build a secure, happy home.
A woman at thirty. My young now grow fast
Bound to each other with ties that should last.
At forty my young sons, near grown, will be gone.
But my man stays beside me to see I don't mourn.
At fifty, once more babies play 'round my knee,
Again we know children, my loved one and me.
Dark days are upon me: my husband is dead.
I look to the future and shudder with dread.
For my young are all busy, rearing young of their own
And I think of the years and the love I have known.
I'm an old woman now, and nature is cruel; it's
Her jest to make old age look like a fool.
The body—it crumbles. Grace and vigor depart.
There now is a stone where I once had a heart.
But inside this old carcass, a young girl still dwells,
And now and again my battered heart swells,
I remember the joys, I remember the pain.
And I'm living and loving life all over again.
I think of the years, all too few—gone too fast
And accept the stark fact that nothing can last.
So open your eyes, nurses! Open and see
Not a crabbit old woman; look closer! See *me*!

—Anonymous

*   This poem was found among the effects of a patient who died at the Oxford University Geriatric Service in England. The author is unknown.

4

Mental Disorders of the Elderly

Objectives

After completing this chapter, the student should be able to:

● appreciate the difficulties of distinguishing the effects of degenerative processes in the brain from the effects of depression, social rejection, and so on
● offer psychological support to the aged
● help orient the confused patient

The type of mental disorder that an elderly person may have and its severity are critical in determining the treatment he will receive. Two general categories of mental disorder exhibited by geriatric patients are:

1. Organic, with evidence of brain damage.
2. Functional, with no evidence of brain damage. Functional disorders can happen to anyone at any age.

Organic Brain Disorders

Organic disorders are associated with cell loss or cell dysfunction. Some neurological deficits resulting from organic brain disorders are: *

Acalculia. Loss of a previously possessed facility with arithmetic calculation.

Agraphia. Loss of a previously possessed facility for writing.

Aphasia. Loss of a previously possessed facility of language comprehension or production that cannot be explained by sensory or motor defects or diffuse cerebral dysfunction.

Apraxia. Loss of a previously possessed ability to perform skilled motor acts that cannot be explained by weakness, abnormal muscle tone, or elementary incoordination.

Confabulation. Fabrication of stories in response to questions about situations or events that are not recalled.

Perseveration. Tendency to emit the same verbal or motor response again and again to varied stimuli.

Reversible organic brain dysfunction is called *acute brain syndrome.* Irreversible dysfunction is called *chronic brain syndrome.*

Acute Brain Syndrome

This temporary mental impairment is often related to malnutrition, infection, small strokes, or medications. The most common symptom is confusion. The patient may also be agitated, panicky, and have hallucinations. When the cause of the syndrome is removed, the patient again becomes normal.

Chronic Brain Syndrome

This disorder is irreversible. The patient is confused as to time, place, and person. There is memory loss for both past and recent events. Judgment is poor and the patient is emotionally unstable.

---

* *This list is from* Aging and Mental Health, *by R. Butler and M. Lewis, pp 78-79, C.V. Mosby, St. Louis.*

The two major causes of chronic brain syndrome are:

1. *Cerebral Arteriosclerosis.* When the cerebral blood vessels thicken and harden, some of the brain's cells are destroyed due to impaired blood supply. Cerebral arteriosclerosis is often first diagnosed after a stroke occurs. However, diffuse brain damage must take place before a person can be labeled as having chronic brain syndrome, and one stroke may not cause that much damage. A person may suffer more than a few strokes before extensive damage occurs. With each individual stroke, however, there may be an episode of acute brain syndrome.

2. *Senile Cerebral Disease.* As Linden states, "Elderly people are frequently regarded as senile by their acquaintances, their families, and even their physicians. Nevertheless, *senility per se* is more a social artifact than a mental disorder."* Senility is an over-used and poorly understood term that has been used to describe certain behaviors apparent in some elderly people. These include altered mental states and what appears to be emotional disorders. It is very difficult to distinguish between disorders caused by mental conflict and disorders caused by brain damage, since the symptoms—depression, nervousness, forgetfulness, and melancholy—are so much alike in both cases.

   Senile cerebral disease (sometimes called "senile psychosis") is caused by atrophy of the brain, which reduces the number of brain cells and increases the size of the ventricles (cavities) in the brain.

   A type of x-ray called computerized axial tomography (CAT) has been helpful in showing the size of the ventricles of the brain. When the brain atrophies, the ventricles become enlarged. Periodic metric evaluations, which are tests in which brain responses are observed by using EEG and selected stimuli, also promise to spot incipient senility.

---

* *Maurice E. Linden, M.D. "Retirement and the Elderly Patient," an address at American Geriatrics Society 32nd Annual Meeting, Miami Beach, Florida, April 16-17, 1975.*

Functional Mental Disorders

Elderly people can be quarrelsome, restless, negative, depressed, agitated, paranoid, or angry. Concealed, untreated depression can become chronic and may result in suicide. Often depressed old people are sure they are becoming senile and this intensifies their depression. It should never be assumed that an old person with a behavioral disorder has brain damage until a definitive diagnosis has been made.

People who are not brain damaged are often called senile if they exhibit depression, forgetfulness, or confusion. These symptoms can have *psychological* causes, including grief for dead loved ones and isolation. Isolation can be geographic, as when children live far away from an aged parent, or it can be physiologic, as when a person has a hearing impairment. Incidentally, hearing impairments can cause effects that are as profound as geographic isolation.

Confusion

Sometimes people seem confused when their problem is really impaired eyesight or hearing, or a slowing of their reaction time. Changes in environment, reaction to restraints, or hospitalization can also bring about confusion, as can drugs, hypoxia, fever, malnutrition, or fluid and electrolyte imbalance.

Depression

It's 11 AM and Mrs. Allen is still in bed. She lies in the fetal position. She hasn't had a decent meal in several days, nor has she dressed herself or stepped out of her room. Every time someone opens her door, she seems to be asleep.

Mrs. Allen is 85 and slightly hard of hearing, but she's not senile. She lives in a nursing home, but she's not sick. In fact, she can care for herself and is economically independent. A nurse asks her what is troubling her and she replies: "I'm not sure. I have no pain, but I don't want to move out of this bed. I'm all right if I lie still. To tell you the truth, I really don't know *what* I want—and I don't care. Why should I bother to get up and get dressed? There's nothing here for me; there's no one I can even talk to. It's just not worth the effort."

A look at Mrs. Allen's background reveals the following information. She has a married son, a wealthy, successful businessman, who visits infrequently though he lives less than two miles away from her. Her daughter is also married and well-to-do, and lives several hundred miles away. Communication between mother and daughter is better than between mother and son, but distance is an inhibiting factor. Last but not least, Mrs. Allen is a widow.

You may have already guessed that Mrs. Allen is depressed. As Butler and Lewis note: "Depression is the most common of the neuroses found in older people. The usual indicators of the presence of depression are feelings of helplessness, sadness, lack of vitality, loneliness, boredom, anorexia . . . . The elderly must deal with their guilt from the past particularly during the life review process through which they examine past actions."

Mrs. Allen exhibits some of the classic symptoms of depression: lethargy (she sleeps a lot); loss of interest (she hasn't dressed, nor has she left her room for several days); anorexia (she's not eating); boredom ("there's nothing here for me"); and helplessness ("I really don't know what I want").

The so-called "golden years" aren't so golden for many aged persons. They lose their spouse and friends, and their children grow up and move away. Moreover, the elderly often lose their purpose or their role in life. People retire and lose their identity with their job. The "empty nest" syndrome causes many women to feel unwanted.

Psychiatrists treat more elderly persons for depression than for any other mental health problem.

Alcoholism, Drug Dependence, Suicide

The Subcommittee on Aging and the Committee on Labor and Public Welfare have conducted research that shows that of the 21 million Americans over 65, possibly 1.6 million are alcoholics. The National Council on Alcoholism ranks alcoholism as a major threat to the health of Americans, right along with cancer and heart disease. A significant number of these 1.6 million elderly people are reactive alcoholics—that is, they started to drink late in life as a reaction to the tragic consequences of being old.

Many gerontologists feel that much of the blame must be laid on a society which is totally preoccupied with youth and regards old age as some sort of disease to be treated.

Drug dependence is a complex problem. Often it is caused by ambivalent physicians. Alcoholism and drug abuse receive scant attention in medical schools, and doctors who become impatient, discouraged, or feel helpless when dealing with geriatric patients may write prescriptions when they probably shouldn't. A deputy assistant commissioner in a Department of Mental Health describes the problem as "poly-pharmacy." Medications that have been tested and approved for younger adults are not tested for use by aged patients. Elderly people have slower metabolic rates and they do not react to medication as do young or mature adults. Moreover, the elderly patient most likely has several ailments he's being treated for, and mixing drugs can cause toxic, even fatal, reactions.

At the Institute of Gerontology of the University of Michigan, researchers claim that people over the age of 65 fall into a high-risk category of mental health problems. While the elderly make up less than 11 percent of the total population, they account for 25 percent of the nation's suicides.

While depression, drinking, and suicide are seen in both aged women and men, more over-65 men than women commit suicide.

Treating Mental Disorders

Psychotherapy, medication, and a range of other methods help geriatric patients with mental disorders. Good management depends on "what can be treated" and "what works." Not too much can be done for the damaged thought centers of the brain, but the patient's mood and behavior can be improved.

Psychotherapy
Disorders associated with mild to moderate brain damage, and depression, alcoholism, and drug addiction may improve with in-

dividual psychotherapy. Group therapy has been found to be useful in increasing patients' self-esteem. These techniques, however, have limited value when the patient has severe organic brain syndrome.

Treatments for Senile Cerebral Disease

A controversial treatment for senility is the use of a hyperbaric chamber. This chamber raises the pressure of oxygen above atmospheric pressure. This oxygen is thought to permeate the brain more efficiently than oxygen at ordinary pressure and to make the patient more alert.

In some cases, blood thinners, which permit blood to pass through clogged arteries have produced desirable effects in terms of alertness and awareness.

Still under investigation is evidence that a chemical substance that accumulates within brain cells contributes to brain aging. The origin of this substance is uncertain but it is associated with slower metabolism, so perhaps a sluggish metabolism encourages its production.

Psychotropic Drugs

There is no one drug that produces a uniform behavioral change in patients. Doctors often have to try various drugs before finding appropriate ones for a patient. Since the body's mechanisms for distributing, detoxifying, and eliminating drugs may be impaired in elderly persons, they may experience more side effects from drugs than younger persons would. To help avoid potential side effects, smaller doses of the drug are usually administered. Because it has been suggested that even mild fear and agitation can bring on or intensify illness, patients experiencing these emotions probably could benefit from tranquilizers. Mild analgesics also help alleviate anxiety by relieving pain.

All nurses are responsible for knowing the drugs their patients are taking and the relationship between the drugs, the diagnoses, and the symptoms presented. Psychotropic drugs are so frequently used with the elderly that the student should know these categories and be able to link them with the symptoms (see table).

Indications for Psychotropic Drugs

Symptoms	Drugs
Frightened, argumentative, or demanding behavior Somatic symptoms Hypochondriasis	Minor tranquilizers and sedatives (e.g., chlordiazepoxide, diazepam, meprobamate, barbiturates); Antihistaminics (e.g., promethazine, chlorpheniramine maleate)
Subjective depression with retardation, agitation	Sympathomimetic stimulants (e.g., amphetamines and methylphenidate); Antidepressants (e.g., tricyclics and MAO inhibitors)
Subjective elation, hypomanic and manic behavior Excitement Delusions Hallucinations	Antipsychotic drugs: phenothiazines (e.g., chlorpromazine); butyrophenones (e.g., haloperidol); and lithium carbonate (specific for mania, hypomania)

Depression, Alcoholism, Drug Abuse

Depression can be treated by psychotherapy, medications, and/or electroshock therapy. Alcoholism and drug abuse require a concerted effort by the medical profession, family, friends, church, and the addicted person himself.

Suicide

Suicide prevention presents special problems. Few elderly take advantage of mental health treatment programs. Pride, misunderstanding, and ignorance are partly to blame. On the other hand, there is a deficiency in many mental health agencies in that they either cannot or do not make the special efforts necessary to seek out the elderly.

How Nursing Staff Can Help

Patients in nursing homes can be helped a good deal if those who are caring for them understand their special problems. Among these are:

    1. Slower reaction time (pace)

2. Dislike of change and a liking for routine
3. The need for self-esteem

Pace

Elderly people have slower reaction times. When they are hurried, they feel reluctant, frustrated, or anxious. A calm, unhurried manner on the part of the nurse or aide will generate trust and cooperation. Coax and encourage elders, and allow them enough time to respond appropriately to your requests.

Change

Elderly people got to *be* elderly by coping successfully with change. Wars, depressions, births, and deaths all were changes they survived. Now that they are elderly, however, they may not react well to change. There is security in structure and routine, whether one lives in one's own home or in a long term care facility. For example, bedtime rituals are common: saying prayers, using certain covers or pillows, and raising or lowering the window.

Sometimes a change that seems right and good can cause serious emotional harm. A prime example is a move. When an elderly parent is widowed, often the children feel that it is wise for him or her to sell the family home and move into something small that is easier to care for. On the surface, the idea seems to have merit. Maintenance is costly and tiring. The property will bring a good price, and so on. But beware. Selling the family home can cause depression and anxiety in the parent and guilt in the child who suggested it. It's not a foolproof solution.

Need for Self-Esteem

Many times health care personnel talk over, around, and about their patients rather than *to* them. Conversation doesn't have to be lengthy. A cheerful greeting, a remark about the weather, a smile, or a friendly touch on the arm all communicate interest. Saying, ''Good morning, Mr. Ryan,'' with eye contact, will raise his feeling of self-worth several degrees.

Treating old people as children fosters childish behavior and regression, not progression. A mark of good nursing care is to promote independence in patients.

Reality Orientation

In a broad sense, reality orientation means continually orienting the confused patient to his identity, to his location, and to the time, and encouraging him to interact with others. The first reality orientation program was organized in the late 1950s in a Kansas Veterans Administration Hospital by James C. Folsom. It was suggested that most of the work be done by attendants, since they spend more time with patients than anyone else. However, it should be used by everyone who comes in contact with confused geriatric patients, especially those who have been institutionalized a long time or who have moderate to severe organic brain impairment.

Folsom organized classes that consisted of no more than four patients to an instructor, who was usually an attendant. The original facts taught were the patient's name, his location, and the date. New facts (age, home town, former occupation) were not introduced until the patient relearned the three basic facts. However, the Do's and Don'ts listed here should be followed all the time by staff personnel. Set routines, consistency, and sincere, friendly interest provide the best foundation for effective reality orientation.

Do's and Don'ts of Reality Orientation*

Do's

1. Do set a routine and stay with it.
2. Do call the patient by his correct name and title (Mr. Smith) unless he specifically asks you to use his first name.
3. Do look at the person you are speaking to; make eye contact.
4. Do reinforce orientation through the use of clocks, calendars, and written reminders (writing in color helps because it is attention grabbing).
5. Do carry on conversations about familiar subjects.
6. Do initiate simple activities, such as brushing teeth or combing hair, that require purposeful movement.

* Adapted from the reality orientation program at the Veterans' Administration Hospital, Tuscaloosa, Alabama.

7.   Be consistent.
8.   Be honest. (Two elderly ladies were sitting side by side in the lounge of a large nursing home. One had had a stroke and was paralyzed. However, she understood what was going on around her and, with difficulty, could speak. The other lady, who had organic brain syndrome, sat rocking in her chair and crying for her mother. No matter how the attendants tried to pacify her, she would not stop crying. With a great effort, the stroke patient said to her, ''I think your mother passed away and I'm sure she's in heaven. Don't you think she's in heaven?'' To everyone's surprise, the crying stopped. Confused people have shown remarkable ability to cope with the truth.)

Don'ts

1.   Don't rush. (Especially, don't push wheelchairs fast—it makes patients dizzy.)
2.   Don't give patients involved tasks to do.
3.   Don't give complicated instructions.
4.   Don't become impatient or discouraged. Allow patients time to answer your questions or to do what you ask.
5.   Don't fail to repeat, over and over if necessary, instructions or basic information.
6.   Don't agree with a confused person's incorrect statements. Gently correct them.
7.   Don't forget to encourage independence in whatever small way you can.
8.   Don't underestimate the importance of touch. It's the most positive means of communication we have and sometimes it's the only means.

Creative Aging

Many people, of course, age creatively. Picasso painted at the age of 90. Leopold Stokowski was recording in his ninth decade and Henry Moore, now in his eighties, still does monumental sculptures. At 80, Verdi composed what many regard as his greatest opera—''Falstaff.'' And, of course, the bubbling Eubie

Blake, the king of ragtime whose life is the story behind "Eubie!," the Broadway musical review, is 95 and still composing.

While these people are certainly impressive, they are greatly outnumbered by lesser known elderly citizens who have continued to be creative in old age. In Aspen, Colorado, a retired 72-year-old pilot devotes his time to teaching the blind to ski. He also spearheaded the founding of BOLD, the Blind Outdoor Leisure Development program. Santa Monica, California, has a 90-year-old talk show hostess who's been involved in radio broadcasting for over 50 years. Henry Washburn, the 68-year-old director of the Boston Science Museum spent four and a half years working with his wife on a detailed map of the Grand Canyon. Over ten million copies of the map have been published. You can probably come up with your own example of an elderly person who is busy and involved with living.

It's very likely that all of these people have some chronic ailment. That's hard to avoid when one reaches the eighth or ninth decade. But they are *doing*, not just *being*.

A poignant story is told about Carl Sandburg. The study where he wrote many poems and his six-volume biography of Lincoln was on the second floor of his home. In his last illness, when

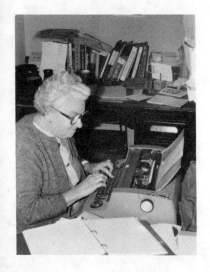

At 73, the author's mother is still employed full time as a "girl Friday" at a small lithographer's plant. She also plays the violin in two amateur symphony orchestras and is active in several church organizations.

he was 89, he insisted on trying to go up the stairs to the study one more time. He crawled on his hands and knees—but he couldn't do it. The last sentence of his own autobiography explains his philosophy: ''If it can be done, it is not a bad practice for a man of many years to die with a boy's heart.'' Sandburg's failure to get up the stairs was unimportant. What did count was the fact that he tried.

DISCUSSION QUESTIONS

1. Think of an elderly person you know. How has he or she adjusted to old age? List the losses this person has endured. What qualities do you think has aided this person to survive so long?
2. What is the main difference between acute brain syndrome and chronic brain syndrome?
3. What are some symptoms old people exhibit that lead to their being erroneously labeled ''senile''?
4. How can impaired hearing or impaired vision lead to confusion?
5. What are some causes of depression in the elderly?
6. What are some ways of encouraging independence in a confused elderly person?

5

The Aphasic Patient

Objectives

After completing this chapter, the reader should be able to:
- understand the causes of aphasia
- understand how therapists work with aphasics to help them relearn language
- help aphasics and their families

Imagine the extreme frustration of the aphasic stroke patient. His intellect is usually normal, but he is unable to communicate his most basic thoughts. Is it any wonder that this patient may become irritable, excited, and even aggressive when he finds that, although he thinks clearly, he has no way of communicating his thoughts and needs?

Caregivers must be continually on guard not to equate aphasia with mental deterioration. It is important for geriatric nurses to have an understanding of aphasia and of how speech therapists teach aphasics communication so that nurses can more effectively contribute to these patients' good care.

What is Aphasia?

Aphasia is an interference with language processes resulting from brain damage. There is a reduction of available language, which may or may not be accompanied by other specific perceptual or sensorimotor deficits compatible with brain damage. Aphasics have difficulty formulating, comprehending, or expressing meanings; there may be impairment in all three areas. Some aphasics find it hard to read; others are unable to write or understand speech or calculate mathematically or, sometimes, even gesture. Since communication, the sharing of information, is a fundamental human activity, impaired communication leads to frustration, anxiety, fear, and a host of negative reactions.

In adults, the most common causes of aphasia are strokes caused by hardening of the arteries, blood clots which block off the nourishing of the nerve cells in the brain, or hemorrhages of the blood vessels in the brain. Other causes are trauma due to auto accidents, brain surgery for tumors, gunshot wounds, and so on.

Prognosis

Immediately after the injury, the patient appears extremely helpless and damaged. Within three or four months, this may subside and what is called "spontaneous recovery" may occur. This is seldom complete, however, and residual aphasia can often be found even in those who have apparently become well.

Spontaneous recovery is rarely seen after six months, and any improvement after this length of time is probably due to the efforts of the patient who is trying to relearn skills and of the therapist who is teaching them to him/her.

Each patient is assessed individually but, in general terms, prognosis is affected by the age, intelligence, and motivation of the patient. Often the attitude of the family, friends, nurses, and doctors create an *unfavorable* prognosis besides contributing to the monumental frustration, depression, and defeatism of the stroke patient.

With professional speech therapy and the cooperation of all who come in contact with the patient, many aphasics regain most of their ability to communicate. Because the nurse should know what the speech therapy consists of so she can reinforce it in her contacts with aphasic patients, a brief summary of it is presented here.

Treatment

Patterns of disability vary widely from case to case. Generally, concentration on the functions *least* impaired is recommended so as to inspire hope in the aphasic. Let him see progress. The general language disability is recognized and improvement aimed for in all areas. The therapist begins and ends each session with things the patient can do. Attempts are made very early in the illness to teach basic communication skills, e.g., how to call for the nurse, how to ask for water, and how to say hello, goodbye, yes, and no.

Parallel Talking

All who speak to the patient should speak clearly and simply. The use of gestures and written and pictured materials at times is very helpful. Therapists practice parallel talking, that is, they tell the patient what is he doing, feeling, or perceiving in simple short sentences or phrases. Often the patient will join in and say a word the therapist is "fumbling" for. It's a basic part of therapy, but it has to be done well. The therapist must know when to hesitate, and it has to be at *exactly* the right moment that the patient is experiencing the thought that the therapist "fumbles" to express. It's also important not to overreact when the patient says the correct word. Just agree and then repeat what the patient has said in the context of the entire statement.

Stimulation

The aphasic lives in a confusing world. Depending on which function is affected, the newspaper seems to be pages of obscure hieroglyphics; he recognizes a clock, but can't tell time. His wife may be talking to him, but he doesn't understand her. He asks her for a glass of water, but she hears only unintelligible jargon.

The speech therapist must first identify what the patient *can* do. For example, can he copy the letters of the alphabet? If not, can he trace over them? Together they will begin at some level he can function at and practice it until the skill is comfortable for the patient. The therapist will try other stimulation. She may have him repeat a sound, a word or a gesture. Together they may each butter a piece of bread. She will take his hand and touch his ear, knee, and the table with it saying the names as she does this. The therapist might have the patient lipread "4" as she places 4 pennies on the table and then have him count to four aloud.

In each session the therapist will review the stimulation, praise success and treat failure matter-of-factly. Success comes as the aphasic's confusion decreases and the lost functions begin to return.

Inhibition

Brain injuries make it difficult to curb emotional outbursts. Laughing, crying, and even tantrums are often observed. The patient may persevere too long. For example, he may start a sentence with "I want" and then, like a broken record, repeat it over and over, being unable to actually tell what it is he wants. The patient needs to be trained to inhibit himself; to stop what he is doing, first at the direction of the therapist and ultimately on his own. The aphasic should practice silently, or with a mirror, or learn to pantomime what he wants.

A therapist will even use "inhibition cards" for patients who can read, The message might be "WAIT," or "STOP LAUGHING," or "WHISPER FIRST!"

Translation

This means training the aphasic to change from one type of symbolism to another. For instance, he will listen to the sound of a cat meowing on a tape recorder. Then the therapist will ask him to identify and spell the name of the animal he heard and then to write (or print) the name of the animal. The object is to give the patient experience in shifting from one set of symbolic meanings to another.

Memorization
Aphasics may be asked to memorize a sequence of movement. This may be an exercise or picking out several objects in a definite order. For example, the therapist may give the patient a catalog and ask him to pick out three items in the order in which they are written on a blackboard. Or the patient's name will be spelled out in block letters on a table and then scrambled so that he has to rearrange them to spell the name correctly. Finally, the patient will be required to memorize prose and poetry. This helps to reinforce word associations and also reviews the basic structure of language.

Scanning and Concentrating
An aphasic may be compared to a man who accidently lands on another planet. Sights and sounds are foreign, even overwhelmingly so. Basic tools and implements used by the natives are mysterious. He must observe and scan for meanings, but he needs the therapist's help. Together they will bring order out of confusion. For example, she may give him a magazine and have him point out all the hats. She will then ask him to stop her every time she says a word beginning with "h." She will have him connect the hat pictures with his own hat. They are selecting and classifying skills most of us take for granted but that have to be relearned by the aphasic.

Organization
The words "scrambled," "jumbled," "confused," and "chaotic" have been used liberally to describe the world of the aphasic. He needs routines, schedules, and structure. The therapist begins with very basic pattern training. The patient may be asked to stack a series of boxes in graduated sizes. Maybe he has to be taught how to set the table or turn the pages of a book from right to left. Together, therapist and patient may sing old, familiar songs. All the planned activities require concentration and scanning by the patient and parallel talking by the therapist.

Formulation
Often the aphasic can't find the words he needs and he is overwhelmed with such depression that he stops right there. He needs

direction and encouragement to try a new and different way which makes sense. Parallel talk and self-talk can help him find verbal symbols that elude him. The following excerpt from a speech therapy session shows how this is done*:

Therapist: All right, John. Let's begin. Talk to yourself. Say what you do. Like this. [She opens her purse, takes out a pencil, and writes his name. As she does so, she speaks in unison with her activity. "Open purse . . . here pencil . . . write name." The therapist hands him the purse and signals him to repeat her behavior.]

John: [Opens purse] 'Oen puss . . . no . . . poos . . no . . . oh dear, oh my . . . . ' [gives up].

Therapist: OK. You got mixed up on purse . . . purrse . . . Never mind. Say the whole thing. [She repeats action]

John: Open puss . . . .

Therapist: And here pencil . . . .

John: Pencil . . . and now I write mame . . . no . . . mama . . . no

Therapist: Write   name . . . name . . . like   this. [Demonstrates]

John: Write name like . . . [writes "John"] . . . John . . . John . . . write no good.

Therapist: Fine! You did it! Now, let's do it again. Talk to yourself. Say what you're doing.

Nurses and family members can describe the activities of daily living in this way and soon the patient will parallel talk as he observes the behavior of others. But this is only the beginning. He has to learn to make change, do mental problems, or, if that's not possible, do simple problems on paper. The aphasic will also be asked to write simple sentences and to write what he is about to say before he says it.

*   *Excerpt from speech therapy session taken from* Speech Correction Principles and Methods, *by Charles VanRiper, Prentice-Hall Inc., Englewood Cliffs, N. J., 1963, p. 453.*

Body Image Integration

If the patient feels as if he has landed on another planet when he is confused by the strange sounds and sights caused by aphasia, he also wonders if his skin has been invaded by an alien. He is not now who he used to be. The family and health care professionals often reinforce this by treating him as if he were a child. An understanding of the situation can prevent this from happening.

What must it be like to find out that overnight one has an arm or a leg or a tongue that won't obey commands? The patient has to be reintroduced to his body all over again. While giving range of motion, the nurse can name the parts of the body she's working with. When teaching lip and tongue movement, it's helpful to use a mirror. A numb hand can be stimulated by massaging it with raw rice. A good therapist and good nursing care can accelerate body image integration.

Psychotherapy

The catastrophic effect of stroke can't be underestimated. The anxieties about money, jobs, and family responsibilities can be overwhelming and certainly are a legitimate reason for psychotherapy. Many therapists feel that a well adjusted person who becomes aphasic has a better chance of ultimate adjustment than a neurotic individual who becomes aphasic. They caution about the problem of psychotherapy with a person who can't communicate. It's extremely difficult to treat someone who can't tell you what he understands or doesn't understand. Often a trial period of therapy is the only way to approach the situation.

How the Nurse Can Help

Patience is an essential component of the nursing approach to the aphasic patient. Speak slowly and allow enough time for your patient to respond. Use nonverbal communication such as gestures and touch. Above all, *talk* to these patients even when they don't respond.

Suggestions You Can Give the Family of the Aphasic Patient

1. *Seek good professional assistance.* The regular advice of a physician is best. The aphasic may need diagnostic tests, medications, nutritional advice and prescribed exercises. Trained social workers, psychologists, and psychiatrists are helpful when there are emotional problems. Remind the family, however, that others besides the skilled team can help the patient recover. Most aphasics improve because of their affectionate support systems, i.e., the family.

2. *Discover how well the patient can communicate.* While diagnostic studies will be used to determine the aphasic's ability, the family should observe the patient's language or lack of it, also. How does the aphasic communicate? Can he gesture? Can he express thoughts, ideas? Efforts to study this will help a person understand what the therapist is doing and ultimately will benefit the patient.

3. *Take a good look at your own feelings.* Aphasia affects the family profoundly. Reactions vary from anxiety and being too helpful to being discouraged and resentful. All these feelings are natural, but they must be recognized. Sometimes an objective, uninvolved third party such as a physician, a clergyman, or a psychologist can be helpful.

4. *Spend time with the patient when he is most responsive.* Aphasics feel isolated because of the severity of their communication problem. Most family members encourage visits with old friends, but it's important to realize that the patient tires easily. During the recovery period, gradually increasing the length of visits is a sensible approach to including the patient in social interaction. The patient's motivation and response will be at a high level *only* if he's rested, so company will be welcome at appropriate times during the patient's daily schedule.

5. *Make a check list of his special interests and use material from it when you spend time with him.* The patient's special interests are as different as each patient is from another. Sports, hobbies, favorite foods—any and all activities form a basis for stimulating the patient. The aphasic's reactions and attitudes have to be closely watched and endeavoring to in-

terest him can be a hit or miss affair. If the response is unfavorable, discard the idea and try something else. Change the subject or just leave the patient alone if he seems upset or restless.

6. *Accept him as he is at the moment.* Outbursts of temper are common. A relaxed, matter of fact attitude is important here because the patient has less control over his emotions than he had before the illness. Be encouraging but avoid false optimism and cliches.

7. *Use every opportunity to increase his independence.* The patient can actually be held back if people do too much for him. The family should aim for daily *small* successes in feeding, dressing, and other activities. They should encourage gains and minimize losses.

8. *Include him in family affairs.* It's irritating to be talked about as if you are not even present. Worse, it's demeaning. Provide for the participation of the patient in conversations, decisions, and activities as much as possible and within reason.

DISCUSSION QUESTIONS

1. What are the causes of aphasia other than strokes?
2. Give examples of nonverbal communication as related to the activities of daily living.
3. What are some ways the nurse can help the family of the aphasic patient?
4. What are some ways the nurse can help the aphasic patient?

6

Sexual Aspects of Aging

by Nancy A. Callahan, RN, BSN, Clinical Supervisor, Medical and Pediatrics, and Instructor, Maternal and Child Nursing, Baystate Medical Center, Springfield, Massachusetts

Objectives

After completing this chapter, the student should be able to:
- understand how normal physiological processes cause changes in the sexual organs of elderly people
- appreciate how the negative attitudes of others may affect sexual behavior in older persons
- help older persons retain their sense of self-esteem

Most honest people will admit that sexuality is one of the most interesting of all human subjects. Curious, then, is the fact that until quite recently the sexual aspects of aging received little attention from researchers or health professionals. Our culture still rejects, to a great extent, the idea that sex is normal and healthy in the later years. It's possible that we have avoided studying this important aspect of aging because professionals also believed that sexual feelings and behaviors did not exist for most of the aging.

What has been learned in recent years can however, help nurses assist the aging to continue to enjoy their sexuality, thus enhancing the quality of their lives.

Age-Related Changes

Masters and Johnson's classic work, *Human Sexual Response,* gave us our first knowledge about the changes in anatomy and physiology of the sexual organs and our first insights into how aging affects sexual response patterns. Since then, other studies have augmented this original work but have not disagreed with the original conclusions. While there are circumstantial and emotional factors which may cause an aging person to refrain from sexual intercourse, there are no inherent physical changes in the aging process of the healthy person which negate sexual behaviors or orgasm.

Changes in Women

Changes in the woman's sexual organs seem to be related primarily to the loss of estrogen production after menopause. Lower estrogen levels cause a loss of elasticity and a thinning of the mucous membranes of the vagina. Consequently, the older woman experiences slower lubrication during sexual excitement than the premenopausal woman. Masters and Johnson found that women who were participating in regular sexual activity, regardless of age, maintained their ability to lubricate better than those who chose not to engage in sex. Also, women who take replacement hormones will experience a more gradual change in vaginal mucosa. Those women who find their lack of lubrication makes penetration uncomfortable can be advised to use a water soluble gel to compensate for nature's lack.

While vaginal changes are to be expected, the clitoris, the major organ of sexual excitation, retains its high degree of sensitivity throughout life. Other characteristic physiological responses to sexual stimulation may diminish (breast changes, skin flushing, uterine contractions) as a woman ages but not enough to interfere with pleasure. Many of the changes of aging go unnoticed by the woman whose sexual life remains vigorous and satisfying.

Changes in Men

The man also experiences changes as he ages but he, too, can rest assured that the changes are of degree, not kind. Testosterone levels gradually decrease with age, causing characteristic physical changes and changes in the timing of sexual response. The older man usually finds that erection takes longer to achieve but he is able to maintain it longer. This aspect of aging is particularly welcomed by the couple disturbed during their younger years by premature ejaculation. The older man also experiences less urgency about ejaculation than his younger counterparts—in fact he often enjoys intercourse without the need to ejaculate. Lower levels of sex hormones diminish the response of the man's nipples, scrotum, and testes to sexual excitement and orgasm. Men experience longer periods of time between erections as they age and some have difficulty re-attaining a "lost" erection during an act of intercourse. The man who is unfamiliar with these expected changes may fear he has become impotent and put aside his sexual life prematurely and unnecessarily.

For both man and woman, then, the physical changes caused by the decline of sex hormone production do not seem to change the capacity for sexual response significantly. It has been reported, however, that the number of sexual encounters lessens as one ages in America. What might account for this if physical changes are not the cause?

Factors Influencing Sexual Choices

Several factors have been discussed in research literature and cited by older persons themselves as influencing their decrease in sexual activity. Some of these are:

Negative attitudes about sex
Chronic illness
Fear of heart attack
Medication side effects
Overindulgence in food or alcohol

Exhaustion

Loss of the usual partner through death or other separation

Lack of opportunity to meet new partners

Loss of self-esteem

Depression

Some of these factors are personal, some circumstantial, some social. A few are beyond the control of either the nurse or the client while others can be prevented or modified. We will consider them individually to see if we as nurses can have a positive role in changing these inhibiting factors.

Negative Attitudes

How and if an older person continues to express sexual needs is often related to cultural beliefs and previously learned expectations. Most of our present older generation grew up in an era of sexual silence, an era in which great gaps in sexual knowledge existed. When gaps in knowledge exist, humans tend to invent answers. With time and repetition, such "answers" become accepted as truth. Some of the "truths" about sexuality prevalent in the early 1900's which still affect the attitudes of older persons are: "nice" women don't experience sexual excitement; sexual interest beyond a certain age (for either sex) is perverse at worst and abnormal at best; marriage and sex should be linked; sex is for reproduction only; and masturbation causes physical and/or mental illness.

Persons who continue to believe these now-discredited notions may have had feelings of guilt about sex throughout much of their lives. They may actually welcome the changes of aging as a reason to stop psychologically uncomfortable sexual behaviors altogether. We need to accept such a choice with respect while not avoiding our professional responsibility to present better information about normal sexuality to them. Others, however, do not share these repressive attitudes and beliefs, and it is these older persons who can most benefit from information-sharing and counseling with health professionals. It is this group who may need some sexual reeducation in order to fully enjoy all their capacities as they age.

Chronic Illness

Chronic illnesses, such as arthritis, emphysema, and vascular disease, may inhibit some older couples from continuing their sexual activity. When properly treated with medication and physical therapy, however, a couple can often maintain their sexual relationship in spite of illness. Changes in love-making positions which may be less stressful for the affected partner could be of help. Side-lying postures for intercourse are often comfortable for both partners. Chronic diabetes is about the only disease which seems to cause impotence in the aging man. As with any type of serious sexual dysfunction, referral for a thorough evaluation of cause is in order before hope is lost.

Fear of Heart Attack

Fear of heart attack during sexual activity is common among the older generation, particularly among those who have already had coronary difficulties or whose partner has heart disease. It has been shown through research that sexual activity, particularly in familiar surroundings with a familiar partner, is akin to any form of moderate exertion. Older persons need to be informed of this research and reassured that sexual activity and heart attack are not directly related to each other. Counseling about less stressful positions for intercourse may also help, although trying new positions seems to actually increase stress for some couples. The warning signs of increased stress should be taught to all cardiac patients and they should consult with their physician if these signs occur during or shortly after sexual activity.

Medications

We know that certain drugs used in the therapy of hypertension, coronary disease, and chronic depression can cause a loss of sexual desire and/or drug-induced impotence. The older person who must use such drugs should be familiar with their expected side effects and report to their doctor if changes in sexual functioning occur. Sometimes an equally therapeutic agent can be substituted for the one causing the problem.

Food, Alcohol, Rest

Overindulgence in food and alcohol can cause sexual problems for anyone but seems to be particularly troublesome to the older man. Encouraging everyone to enjoy food and drink wisely and to keep a good balance between rest and exercise is a nursing responsibility. The older person who is in good physical condition is more likely to enjoy *everything,* including sex!

Loss Through Death or Separation; Lack of New Partners

Loss of loved ones through death is a sad but common experience for older persons. Saddest of all during the later years may be the loss of one's love partner, for new sexual relationships are often very difficult to establish. Two cultural biases mitigate against the formation of new relationships—the idea that older persons shouldn't be interested anyway and, secondly, the feeling that sex is for married persons only (at least if you're over 60!). Less effort is made by friends and relatives to introduce the older person to potential partners than would be the case for younger widows and widowers. Places where younger people go to meet new people are often unwelcoming and suspicious of older persons. Sons and daughters often have strong feelings against remarriage and extremely negative feelings about any other form of sexual relationship for their parents. Until recently, even the law made it financially unprofitable to remarry after 65. Chances are that persons who lose their sexual partner late in life will spend their remaining years alone.

Another form of separation can be equally devastating to an older, sexually active couple. Circumstances may necessitate the move of one of them from the home to a nursing home or other supervised living situation. While the husband or wife (or lover) will be encouraged to visit, there is hardly ever enough privacy for the intimate relationship to be continued. Semi-private rooms, unlocked doors and staff moving freely in and out are hardly conducive to loving! Even if both partners move to supervised living, they are often separated and given a roommate of their own sex.

Loss of Self-Esteem; Masculinity and Femininity

Probably the greatest inhibitor of healthy sexual functioning in older age is loss of self-esteem and the development of a negative self-image. It is difficult to maintain one's positive self-image in a culture as devoted to youth worship as ours is. Loss of skin and muscle tone, graying hair, wrinkles, and "liver spots" are certainly not revered by Madison Avenue and Hollywood! The attitude that young is beautiful and sexy and that old is not pervades the thinking of many of us.

But being sexual and sexually attractive is more than one's physique—it involves those elusive qualities called masculinity and femininity and doing things which make one feel good about being a man or being a woman. When middle-aged persons were asked what makes them feel successful as a man or a woman, women tended to answer: dressing attractively; smelling good; being a good cook or homemaker; wearing make-up and jewelry; helping others; being a good wife, mother, or daughter; and receiving compliments. Men mentioned such things as: being successful in their work; managing money well; participating in sports and other activities with men; discussing politics and world events knowledgeably; advising younger people; being attractive to women; and being a good lover. (These activities may seem stereotyped to the reader and, in one sense, they are. Many of our older citizens grew up in an era when "masculinity" and "femininity" were more rigidly defined than nowadays.)

When one feels good about oneself and one's self-confidence is high, something is communicated to others which translates into sexual attractiveness, regardless of age. Unfortunately, many of our older citizens live in environments which are not sensitive to the importance of helping them maintain a positive self-image. Premature cessation of those activities which previously built self-esteem, such as dressing attractively or participating in sports, sap the zest from life for them, as it would for us.

Depression

Any of the factors discussed previously may lead to transient or chronic depression in our older clients. Frequently, several of the factors are operating simultaneously in their lives. The depressed person rarely has much energy for any of life's activities, including sexual activity.

What Can the Nurse Do?

In the face of all the possible inhibitors discussed above, the nurse may feel helpless and hopeless about having a positive role in helping older persons continue to enjoy their sexual capabilities! Such hopelessness leads many of us to give up before we should—or avoid the issue entirely! Here are some things I think we *can* do:

● Recognize our own obstructive attitudes about sex among the elderly. It is almost impossible not to have learned some negative attitudes during our own growing-up years. Once we recognize our own attitudes, we can begin the process of reeducation for ourselves as individual practitioners and for the profession as a whole. The new information being generated by research is not only important, it is interesting.

● Acknowledge and respect the continuing sexual needs of the older adult. The tendency to infantilize the elderly may have been one of our unconscious ways of avoiding our own discomfort about sexual expression at their age. Once we recognize and accept them as sexual persons, our relationships with them must change. That very change in our behavior can contribute much to the older person's positive self-image, which in turn will help him or her feel sexually attractive. Occasionally, a client's sexual needs and desires will be directed at the health care professional. While we recognize flirtatious or seductive behavior as inappropriate to a professional relationship, we may find ourselves unable to cope with our own feelings in such situations. We may be tempted to simply avoid further interaction with the client. Gentle reminders about limits or, better yet, an open, frank discussion of their needs and feelings is more productive and caring than avoidance. If the professional feels unprepared to confront inappropriate behaviors alone, the assistance of a supervisor or coprofessional should be sought.

- Help older persons continue those activities which contributed to feelings of masculinity and femininity in their younger years. Here is an opportunity to assess and individualize our nursing care for each client. Once we know what *they* choose for themselves, we can direct our efforts toward providing continuation of similar activities. We may need to provide transportation so that an older client can participate in community affairs or go to the beauty parlor or barber. We need to encourage women to continue cooking (or at least, to share recipes with the cook) and to encourage widowers to learn to cook for their own better nutrition. Opportunities for people to gather together to discuss politics or to watch sporting and other events can be provided in most settings. Other creative approaches will undoubtedly occur to health care professionals once they give priority to the maintenance of the older person's self-image.

- Encourage good physical habits through exercise, rest, and nutrition. Too often, we tacitly encourage older persons to spend most of their waking hours sitting around, which only compounds the natural loss of tone and circulation.

- When a "couple" already exists, provide opportunities for privacy. In some supervised living situations, policies may have to be revised in order to provide an older couple with time alone together. We should beware, however, of assuming that every older couple wants to continue being roommates! It should be their choice, supported by us and reevaluated from time to time. If they do choose to share the same room, using their own bed in the new setting may encourage them to continue already established sexual patterns.

- Provide social outlets and encourage new friendships that may lead to intimate relationships. We are sometimes guilty of treating a newly-forming couple as "cute" and joking about their relationship. Older persons, highly sensitive to criticism and poorly educated about sexuality in old age, will conform to what we are implying, thereby losing valuable opportunities to replace lost partners.

- Refer clients to physicians for health checks-ups (including pelvic exams) and re-evaluation of medications. Pain on intercourse, impotence unrelieved by changes in eating or drinking styles, and chronic depression need a specialist's intervention. The informed, interested doctor is our most valuable collaborator in reeducating our older clients toward healthier living and continued sexual expression. Using his/her authority judiciously, the physician can reinforce the nurse's teaching and counseling and provide reassurance.

- Share new-found information on normal sexual functioning in older persons with clients, families, and professional peers. We cannot hope to accomplish much in a vacuum which continues to repress sexual knowledge and to perpetrate sexual mythology. Fortunately, most persons are interested in knowing more about that ever-fascinating subject of human sexuality! Changing deep-seated attitudes is, of course, difficult and the nurse needs to accept this. It is our responsibility, however, to continue to try to influence persons of all ages towards healthier sexual attitudes and more informed decision-making about their sexuality.

While these nursing activities will not make us qualified sexual therapists, they can add a new dimension to our nursing of older persons and, hopefully, add to the joy of our clients' later years.

DISCUSSION QUESTIONS

1. Suggest ways in which alert people living in nursing homes can be helped to form new relationships.
2. Suggest ways in which healthy elderly people living in the community can be helped to form new relationships.
3. Do you think that there may be some or many elderly people who do not wish to form new relationships and who might resent being pressured to do so?

7

Common Geriatric Nutrition Problems

Objectives

After completing this chapter, the student should be able to:

- understand how nutrition is linked to many medical problems
- realize that finances play an important part in how well elders eat
- be aware that there are psychological reasons why older persons may not eat balanced diets
- know what can cause malnutrition problems in hospitals
- solve some specific nutrition problems

Nutritional Deficiencies

The most rapidly increasing minority in the world today is the over-65 age group. Women outnumber men two to one. Typically, it is a woman over 65, now living alone, who is most likely to be depriving herself of essential nutrients, the nutrients she was careful to see that her family received.

What happened to the housewife who spent long hours cooking cereals, baking bread, and shopping for fresh meats, fruits, and vegetables? The answer can be found in three constantly overlapping components: physical, economic, and psychological.

The Physical Component

Poor nutrition can lead to a number of problems, including:

Heart Disease. The leading cause of death in this country, heart disease strikes men and women indiscriminately, beginning in the peak productive years and continuing through old age. The American Heart Association reveals that a contributing cause is a high intake of calories (mostly those of saturated fat and refined sugar) and a correspondingly low expenditure of energy.

Obesity. This condition is common in postmenopausal women. As we age, our physical activity decreases and so does our basal metabolic rate. If calories aren't trimmed to accommodate this decrease, obesity is the inevitable result. And it's not sufficient just to eat *less.* An obese elderly person presents a complex problem because, if activity can't be increased to help burn up excess calories, then the diet has to be pared down while still allowing for sufficient amounts of calcium, protein, and iron.

Girth control in the elderly is a challenging objective. The rewards include less cardiovascular disability, less discomfort for the arthritic, and increased muscular strength.

Iron-Deficiency Anemia. The most prevalent nutritional deficiency in the elderly is iron-deficiency anemia, probably because high meat prices consume too large a part of the food budget. A lack of green and yellow vegetables in the diet also helps to cause this problem.

Decrease in Muscular Strength. A disturbing number of deaths of persons over the age of 65 are accidental. The most frequent accident is a fall and this is generally because of diminished muscular strength, another example of the interdependence between nutrition and overall health and well-being.

Osteoporosis. This condition, characterized by abnormal pourousness, fragility, and reduction in the quality of bone, is most often seen in women after menopause. Partly due to a disturbance of mineral metabolism, it may also be partly due to an insufficient intake of milk, cheese, and other foods rich in calcium.

Dental Problems.   These loom large as a physical consideration. Nearly one-third of all Americans and two-thirds of those
over 65 have lost all of their natural teeth. By middle age, 25
million people are edentulous; another 25 million have lost half of
their teeth. If dentures don't fit well or haven't had necessary
repairs, chewing becomes difficult or impossible. Mastication is
an essential first step of the digestive process. Deficiencies in this
first step can lead to taking an improper diet which in turn leads to
undernutrition or obesity or various illnesses caused by dietary in-
sufficiencies. The solution seems deceptively simple: sound prophylaxis or at least properly fitted dentures. Unfortunately, many
elderly are on fixed incomes and dental care is costly.

Dry Skin and Decreased Mucus Secretion.   Common in older
people, these conditions may be partly caused by vitamin A deficiency due to a low fat diet.

Polyneuritis.   This inflammation of many peripheral nerves at
the same time can be due to a thiamine deficiency (thiamine is present in whole grain cereals and breads).

Lack of Mobility.   In a sense, lack of mobility may also be
regarded as a physical problem. The elderly adult who can't drive
and can't carry too many parcels has to practice defensive
marketing. Purchases must be economical and lasting. Often that
precludes buying fresh meats and produce. Instead, pastries and
canned goods of limited nutritional value are bought. There are
several ways community services can help. Meals on Wheels
programs insure delivery of one hot meal daily to the elderly person who is unable to cook or to get out and shop. Group shopping
trips also narrow the gap between market and pantry. The federal
government has funded a nutrition program for the elderly under
Title VII of the Older American Act. While administered by different agencies in different states (departments of health or public
welfare), basically all agencies provide a quality diet prepared and
distributed to the elderly at low or no cost in a community facility.

The Economic Component
It is estimated that of the 23 million elderly, 3.3 million live below
the poverty level. The Ten-State Nutrition Survey demonstrates

that as income decreases, the incidence of malnutrition increases. As inflation nudges prices upward, the elderly citizen on a fixed income has severely limited purchasing power. Ironically, the very foods that contain the most important nutrients—protein and calcium—are the most expensive. The survey clearly shows that malnutrition in persons over 65 is caused by poor food choices and lack of money. Social Security is the only source of income for many elderly people. While the benefits have been increased from time to time, it doesn't seem as if these increases will keep pace with inflation.

Of the 3.3 million persons who are elderly and are living below the poverty level, most did not become poor until they became old. Americans are retiring earlier and living longer. The elderly themselves suggest that Social Security regulations be revised to avoid penalizing them for working for money they need in order to support themselves and to purchase the foods they need. Others would like to see business and industry eliminate forced retirement. This goal seems very near. If an employee is capable, why not keep him as a productive, taxpaying citizen (particularly if he doesn't have a sound retirement plan)?

The Psychological Component

Mr. Taylor, 70, lives alone. She's in fairly good health. Her late husband's pension plan, supplemented by Social Security benefits, provide her with an adequate standard of living. For breakfast Mrs. Taylor has toast and coffee; lunch is usually soup or a sandwich. At supper time she may open a can of spaghetti or ravioli. Occasionally she varies this with scrambled eggs. When she forgets to eat lunch or supper, which happens from time to time, she nibbles on pastries, cookies, and now and then a candy bar.

Mrs. Taylor can comfortably afford a more varied, nutritionally sound menu. Why doesn't she include meat, fresh fruits, vegetables, and dairy products in her diet? "When my two children were small, I used to love to cook. In fact, the first thing I did after they were off to school and my husband left for work was to make a special dessert for supper. When the boys grew up and married, I missed them with a real ache. But I still had my husband to fuss over. Now that he's gone, it just doesn't seem worth the trouble to cook for one person."

The loss of role in the family is a determining factor in under-nutrition of the elderly. When Mrs. Taylor was no longer needed as mother and wife she lost part of her identity.

Henry and Ada Marks were childless. When Mrs. Marks died last year, her husband was lost. He barely knew how to use a can opener because his wife had always taken such good care of him. Mr. Marks is a vigorous 69 but he exists on anything that "comes out of a can or box and doesn't need fussing." He's close to a fast food chain and he patronizes it as a matter of convenience a few times a week. How much longer will this man be vigorous on such a limited diet? Lack of knowledge about how to shop and prepare food is a big stumbling block to many elderly, particularly if there's no motivation for learning.

Margaret and Alice Miller are retired school teachers in their late 70's. Margaret has edematous legs secondary to congestive heart failure. She's a semi-invalid confined to the house. Alice tries to take care of the marketing chores, a difficult task for an obese arthritic. She moves slowly and painfully down the five blocks to the supermarket. Once there, she selects ground meat, day-old pastries, and some canned goods. On the return trip she stops at a package store. Alice is alcoholic, and three or four days a week she's in a stupor. Alcoholism, which can be a conse-quence of poor mental health, insecurity, or despair, is a common problem of the malnourished elderly.

Emotionally caused malnutrition isn't limited to a certain social class or income bracket. It can be difficult to motivate some persons to eat properly. Many elderly need to be convinced that money spent for food is money well spent. Others need reinforce-ment of a sense of self-worth.

Eating has social connotations. We join friends for coffee, celebrate with a dinner. Most of us don't like to eat alone because we have always associated some social or family activity with food. This underscores the key role that sharing meals and com-panionship can play in maintaining satisfactory nutrition levels.

According to N. J. Grills, "Most general complaints, i.e., fatigue, apathy, anorexia, nervousness, headache, irritability, dyspepsia, and depression may be a sign of psychogenic originating disease. If nutritionally related, this can be simply and inexpensively relieved by improving the quality and quantity of nutrients. Sometimes symptoms disappear after the elderly are treated with multivitamins for several months.''

That statement is certainly a strong case for developing cooking and marketing skills. Preparing balanced meals need not be a waste of food and money. Most of us would acknowledge that it's not easy to change the eating habits of a lifetime. But it makes sense to accustom ourselves to proper eating so we can avoid illness.

There is no essential change in nutritional needs with advancing age. We may need to take in fewer calories if we become less active, but the consumption of adequate amounts of protein, calcium, and iron, plus other essential nutrients is as important to the septuagenarian as it is to the adolescent.

The Five Most Common Nutrients and How They Act

1. *protein*—builds, preserves, and restores bodily tissue
2. *carbohydrate*—supplies energy and fuel for the body
3. *fat*—supplies twice as much energy and fuel as carbohydrate; also has twice as many calories; contains vitamins A and D
4. *minerals*—essential for bone, teeth, and red blood cell formation
5. *vitamins*—substances necessary for the utilization of food

Most of us don't have to look too far to find an elderly person with a nutrition problem. We may even have one in our own family. Perhaps that person could be helped simply by cooking a little more for the family and then freezing a portion for the grandmother or father-in-law who lives alone. How about helping with their marketing on a regular basis? A better nourished, more vigorous elderly adult is surely worth the extra effort.

Malnutrition in the Hospital

Malnutrition is a serious geriatric problem overlooked by many health care professionals. It isn't limited to Appalachia or the city slums, either. It develops in some of our most modern hospitals.

Hospital admission gives many people a false sense of security. "I'm in good hands," thinks the patient, settling back in bed. "He's getting the best of care," says the family with a collective sigh of relief. The unhappy truth is that malnutrition often flourishes under the noses of health care professionals who either don't know or ignore the fundamentals of their patients' nutritional health.

Agnes Newell, 69, is a patient on an orthopedic unit. She is recovering from a fractured hip. A victim of organic brain syndrome, she had been admitted from the nursing home where she had lived for three years. At mealtimes, a young dietary aide serves her a tray and 45 minutes later two nurses' aides roll a cart down the corridor and swiftly collect all the trays. No one is sure how much Mrs. Lowell eats—or if she eats anything—and she's too confused to tell them.

Leonard Hull, 66, is restrained. He's in the throes of delireum tremens. His IVs, vital signs, and neurological signs are meticulously charted. A closer look reveals pages of physicians' orders, laboratory test results, and x-ray reports. A more detailed work-up would be hard to find. However, there's one important omission: no one has recorded Mr. Hull's height and weight.

Richard Marlow, 75, is in the hospital hoping to learn the cause of his abdominal pain. Yesterday he fasted for an upper GI series. The schedule was delayed, and by the time he got back to his room lunch was over. Today he's having an IVP at noon. He'll miss breakfast and lunch—again.

Leading the list of practices that interfere with or prevent optimum nutritional health for hospital patients are the three incidents that involved Mrs. Newell, Mr. Hull, and Mr. Marlow, i.e., failure to observe and record food intake, absence of recorded height and weight, and failure to provide food after meals are missed because of diagnostic tests. These practices are dangerous and objectionable for the following reasons.

A well adult who consumes between two and three thousand calories daily may need twice that amount when subjected to the stress of surgery and fever. Mrs. Newell is confused and she has had surgery for her fractured hip. While she can feed herself, it is a nursing responsibility to monitor her meals. Hunger will make her uncomfortable and frustrated. But more important, inadequate food intake will also retard her convalescence and ultimate healing.

Alcoholics get most of their calories from alcohol and most of these are "empty calories," nutritionally worthless. Mr. Hull may already be underweight. He will be on IVs for several days and, while these parenteral fluids will hydrate him adequately, they will not supply him with sufficient calories. He's certain to lose more weight, but there's no way to calculate this accurately unless he was weighed upon admission.

Mr. Marlow's problem is different from Mrs. Newell's and Mr. Hull's but it's no less serious. He has never paid much attention to his diet and his normal eating habits are irregular to say the least. In theory, hospitalization should guarantee him nutritionally balanced meals but so far it hasn't worked out that way. He has only "picked at" food that has been served and he has missed several meals because of his test schedule. Now he may need surgery. The caloric cost of that stress plus the nutritional demand in the subsequent cell and tissue repair will put enormous demands on his metabolism that may not be met. The way food substances are broken down and the way new cells are developed can be affected by these combined stress situations. His levels of hemoglobin and plasma protein will drop, as will his red blood count if he isn't consuming a carefully balanced diet. He'll be likely to have muscle weakness, pulmonary problems and cardiovascular insufficiency. In extreme cases, survival depends on the balance between the impact of stress and the mobilization of the body's protective mechanisms, namely, cell metabolism and function. Problems can be prevented when there is protein synthesis sufficient to enable the body to bear the stresses of illness and surgery.

Finding the Causes of Malnutrition

Malnutrition can be dealt with successfully only if health care professionals know how to find its causes. They must accurately assess the present condition of the patient before they can determine why he is poorly nourished. Then they must estimate and supply the calories, proteins, vitamins, and electrolytes that are essential for good nutrition.

The root causes of malnutrition are complex. Sometimes dentures are not fitted properly. Sometimes the patient has difficulty swallowing or digesting food. But in many hospital situations the nurse has some control. Estimating and providing nutrients requires the joint effort of physician, nurse, dietitian, and patient.

Why is the nurse the likely person to become involved with the nutritional state of the patient? Initially, the physician prescribes the diet. The dietitian sees that the order is fulfilled and explains the diet to the patient. The doctor is concerned with the "nuts and bolts" of the patient's physical recovery. He's occupied with blood work, medications, and treatments. The dietitian may have from 75 to 100 patients she's responsible for. Who is in a better position than the nurse to note the patient's height and weight, intake and output, eating habits, and to verify that the patient is getting the right diet? Equally important, the nurse can let the patient know that substitutions are available. The nurse is the valuable reinforcer of the plan for nutritional therapy.

Nutrition is vital to successful therapy and health maintenance. The nurse is the key person to insure that the patient's nutritional needs are met.

Nutritional Assessment Test
How can a patient's nutritional status be assessed if he can't or won't cooperate? Besides measuring height and weight, some hospitals have developed and use nutritional assessment tests. For example, they examine a specimen of blood to check for albumin and total lymphocyte count. Then four intradermal injections are given, two in each arm. The antigens used are monilia, mumps, PPD (purified protein derivative) and SK-SD (streptokinase-streptodornase). Indurations are measured within 48 hours. A triceps skin fold is measured with calipers and a mid-upper arm circumference is taken. The blood test, skin reactions and measurements are compared to a given set of criteria and a nutritional assessment is made based on this information. This unique nutritional profile tells whether a patient is normally nourished, moderately malnourished, or severely malnourished. Treatment is prescribed accordingly. This is a rather new test and

it's inexpensive for the patient. One day it may be as common as a CBC or urinalysis.

Solving Some Nutrition Problems

● PROBLEM: Iron deficiency anemia.

SOLUTION: This can be corrected by adequate intake of protein. While most elderly adults recognize that a hot meal consisting of meat and vegetables is desirable and is a good way of getting protein, not all are aware that there are easy and inexpensive ways to increase the protein value of foods. Here are some ways that this can be done:

Protein Packed Milk

This is actually double-strength milk made by adding one cup of dried milk to one quart of liquid whole milk. (Ordinarily you would add dry milk to water.) One cup of this will provide twice as much protein as whole milk   or skim milk.

Protein packed milk can be flavored by the addition of pureed fruits, fruit syrups, chocolate syrup, vanilla, and so on. It can also be used in cooking, e.g., in soups, cereals, puddings, creamed foods (tuna, chicken), meat loaf, mashed potatoes, and scrambled eggs.

High Protein Milk (one-half cup equals eight grams of protein)

To one quart of whole or skim milk, add one-half cup of skim milk powder. Mix thoroughly and chill. To be used as double-strength milk or taken between meals. There are more calories if it is made with whole milk.

High Protein Egg Nog (one-half cup equals ten grams of protein)

1 quart whole milk   ¼ cup sugar
¾ cup skim milk powder   1 tsp vanilla
2 eggs   nutmeg to taste

Beat eggs. Add whole milk and sugar. Mix well, sprinkle milk powder and flavoring over egg and milk mixture. Beat until smooth (or put all ingredients into a blender). Chill before serving. Serve one-half to three-fourths cup portions between meals. Makes six to eight servings.

More About Protein

The American Dietetic Association recommends .9 gram of protein per kilogram of body weight. Multiply the number of pounds a person weighs by 2.2 to determine the corresponding weight in kilograms.

A woman over the age of 51 requires about 40 grams of protein per day. A man the same age requires about 48.

Sample Foods and Their Protein Content

		Daily Meals
8 oz. milk (whole or skim)	8 grams	8 grams
1 oz. meat, fish, poultry 1 egg 2 tablespoons peanut butter 1 oz. cheese ¼ cup cottage cheese	7 grams	28 grams (4 **servings**)
1 serving starch (grains, cereals, bread)	2 grams	8 grams (4 servings)
½ cup vegetables	2 grams	4 grams (2 servings)
		48 grams

NOTE: If snacks are to be used in daily diets, make them high protein quick snacks. Some examples would be: yogurt, cheese, peanut butter, nuts, luncheon meats, precooked sausage, prepared sandwich fillings.

● PROBLEMS: Obesity, heart disease.
SOLUTION: Low fat, low sodium diets. In addition to reducing caloric intake, a person troubled with obesity will benefit from a low fat diet, i.e., a diet in which the main modification in the nutrient content is that the fat content is reduced. Dairy products are permitted but are limited to skim milk, buttermilk, yogurt, uncreamed cottage cheese and a limited amount of butter or margarine.

Appropriate meats are chicken, turkey, and veal. Fish is permitted.

The low fat diet must be monitored in order to prevent a possible vitamin A deficiency.

A low sodium diet is prescribed in order to prevent edema, an accumulation of water, and sodium in the body tissues that results in a swollen appearance and occurs in cardiovascular disease. The diet isn't 100 percent free of sodium because traces of this element are found in water and most foods. However, by restricting salt, a tolerable sodium level is maintained. Sodium regulates water balance in the body.

A problem with this type of diet may be a lack of flavor. Herbs and mild spices may be used to enhance food tastes.

The following publications are available free from your local Heart Association chapter or from the National Heart Association office:

Save Food $ $ and Help Your Heart, 50-032A
Eat Well but Wisely to Reduce Your Risk of Heart Attack,
     51-005A
A Guide to Weight Reduction, 50-034A

In addition to these publications, free booklets of low-sodium receipts are put out by the Campbell Soup Company. Write to:

Low Sodium, GH Box 288 CC
Collingswood, New Jersey 08108

● PROBLEM: Dental deficiencies.
SOLUTION: Soft diet. When chewing is a problem, whether because of poorly fitted dentures or lack of dentures, it may be necessary to use a soft diet. This type of diet includes finely diced meats or ground meats and pureed fruits or vegetables in addition to a vast number of soft foods — enough to provide a satisfactory variety and a well balanced diet. In fact, the only restrictions are: tough, fibrous meat; whole meat or poultry; whole frankfurters; shrimp, scallops, hard cheeses, hard fried eggs, coarse bread or rolls with seeds, raisins, nuts, and all the raw fruits or vegetables the person can't chew.

● PROBLEM: Constipation.*
SOLUTION: The following suggestions may be used as a guide in encouraging the patient to choose foods that will help correct or avoid constipation.

---

*   *This section on constipation is from* Bowel Evacuation Manual and Bowel Retraining Record, *courtesy of Boeringer Ingelheim Ltd.*

Foods that dietitians refer to as "high residue," "bulky," or "fibrous" are often helpful to the person troubled with constipation. They are not completely used by the body and so they provide bulk in the large intestine. This bulk encourages evacuation.

While fruits and vegetables are often recommended for bulk, not all are useful. If the patient may have high-residue foods, he should be encouraged to select the following items from his menu or tray:

salads of *raw* fruits or vegetables
vegetables with long fibers (greens, kale, cabbage, celery)
whole fruits with skin rather than peeled fruits or juices
stewed prunes, apricots, or figs
dried fruits (apricots, figs, dates, prunes)
cereals and bread with part of the whole grain in them

Whole grain cereals and dark bread provide bulk since the grain covering is not digested by the body. The following foods and menus will help overcome constipation.

Suggested Foods	*Sample Menu*
Breakfast	
fruit	prunes
whole-grain cereal	oatmeal
bacon or egg	2 strips bacon
whole-grain bread	1 slice whole wheat bread
butter	1 pat butter
cream, milk	as needed for cereal
coffee or tea	beverage as desired
Lunch	
soup	vegetable soup
meat, fish, fowl	swiss steak
potato	mashed potatoes
vegetable	beets
salad (fr. or veg.)	gelatin fruit salad
whole-grain bread	1 slice whole wheat bread
butter	1 pat butter
dessert	baked apple with cream
milk, coffee, tea	beverage as desired

Dinner

meat, fish, fowl, eggs	cold meat
potato, rice, macaroni	spanish rice
vegetable	buttered carrots
salad	vegetable salad
whole grain bread	1 slice whole wheat bread
butter	1 pat butter
dessert	tapioca pudding
milk	1 glass milk

Snacks

3 PM, fruit juice

8 PM, fruit juice

If necessary, more vegetables, fruits, and fruit juice may be added.

● **PROBLEM:** Anorexia.*

SOLUTION: Various techniques to encourage oral intake:

1. Patients complaining that foods have lost their taste should be encouraged to experiment with a variety of flavors and *aromas.* Flavoring extracts and a variety of spices enhance the flavor of foods. People can be taught that various food aromas help stimulate appetite and improve mental attitude.

2. Patients experiencing anorexia and early satiety should be advised to eat small, frequent meals.

3. Relatives should be cautioned against developing the "eat a little more" syndrome, and they should be encouraged to create a natural, pleasant atmosphere during meals.

4. Fruit juices or other high caloric beverages can be substituted for coffee, tea, or water.

5. Fresh fruits may make ice cream, milk shakes, puddings, custards, and commercial food supplements more appealing.

6. Between-meal supplements can be encouraged to add to daily protein and calorie intake.

* *Adapted from Ross Laboratories'* Dietary Modifications, *Ross Laboratories Division of Abbott Laboratories, Columbus, Ohio.*

7. Diet should be modified in texture and consistency (bland, soft) to accommodate individual needs.
8. Meticulous oral hygiene should be carried out. Scrupulously clean teeth and mouth enhance the taste of food.

● PROBLEM: Diabetes Mellitus.

SOLUTION: The basis of diabetic therapy is diet and patients should be asked, if feasible, to cooperate in eating correctly. The diet is calculated by using 30 calories per kilogram (2.2 pounds) of body weight when the patient is at his ideal body weight. This diet is adjusted by adding five or ten calories per kilogram more or less if the patient needs to gain weight.

The caloric intake is divided into 40 percent carbohydrate, 40 percent fat, and 20 percent protein. These nutrients are the foundation of the simple food exchange system which divides all foods into four basic exchanges: meat, bread/cereal, fruit/vegetable, and milk groups. For example, one small apple is one fruit exchange, one slice of bread is one bread exchange, and one ounce of meat is one meat exchange.

Basic Four Food Groups

1. *Meat*	2. *Bread/Cereal*	3. *Milk*	4. *Vegetable/Fruit*
meat	bread	milk—whole,	vegetables
poultry	cereal	skim, evaporat-	fruit
fish	macaroni,noodles	ed, dry, butter-	
eggs	and spaghetti	milk, etc.	
peanut butter	rice	cheese, including	
beans		cottage cheese	
		ice cream, yogurt	

The diabetic's diet is controlled by having him eat the same number of calories and the same food exchanges each day. Now, this doesn't mean that a patient must eat the same foods each day. Rather, it means that the patient can't substitute a fruit exchange for a bread exchange.

It's important to design a diet, based on the physician's prescription, that meets the patient's needs, because it isn't

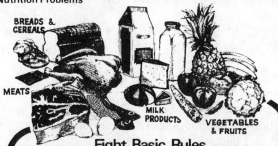

Eight Basic Rules
for Diabetic Food Preparation

1. Understanding the food exchange lists is the key to cooking or selecting delicious foods for the diabetic diet.

2. Spend enough time planning meals. Read your local newspaper ads to keep up with foods in season and those featured at special prices. Plan your meals and your family's meals by the week and shop accordingly. Select your main dish from the meat list on your diet and then choose vegetables, salad, fruit, bread or substitute to go with it.

3. You should not need to buy a great many special diet foods. You will find that you will be able to eat the same meats, vegetables, salads and fruits as your family most of the time. The amount of fat added in preparation should always be considered in your diet. Your neighborhood grocer can supply you and your family with food which is nutritionally adequate in every way. Neither you nor your family needs organically grown foods or other unusual items. If you are eating a variety of foods, you should not need added vitamin supplements. If you have a special need for them, your doctor will suggest one.

4. Provide yourself with good cooking utensils, measuring cup, spoons and possibly scales. You deserve to pamper yourself a little by using a variety of spices and selected seasonings.

5. You may adapt recipes from standard cookbooks to your own eating pattern.

6. You do need to buy good meats, vegetables and fruits. If you are using these foods in the proper amounts and eliminating those you should not use, you may be buying *less* food.

7. Don't tempt yourself by keeping many "forbidden" foods around the kitchen. The better job you do with the diabetic diet, the less they will interest you.

8. A good rule for all "cooks": Remember that an attractive and simple meal served in a happy and congenial family atmosphere is more important to everyone than the number of heavy, overly rich foods served at the table. Children often enjoy their food more if they can sometimes invite a friend to eat it with them or if colorful foods or bright paper plates and napkins are used.

A list of rules for diabetic patients. Courtesy of Monoject.

realistic to give the patient a diet that he absolutely will not follow. The following recipes for diabetics are suggestions.*

Zero Salad Dressing
Tomato juice, ½ cup
lemon juice or vinegar, 2 tablespoons
onion, finely chopped, 1 tablespoon
salt and pepper, to taste
Combine the ingredients in a jar with tightly fitted top. Shake well before using. This dressing may be used in any amount.

Chopped parsley or green pepper, horseradish or mustard, may be added if desired.

Baked Chicken
1 fryer, whole	soy sauce or Worcestershire sauce
salt	celery leaves and pieces

Wash chicken and sprinkle lightly with salt in cavity and on outside. Sprinkle cavity and outside liberally with the sauce. Stuff with celery and leaves. Place in covered roasting pan and bake at 350 degrees at 25 minutes per pound, or until tender. Use only in amounts allowed in diet.

Vegetable Soup for One
1 cup clear meat stock or bouillon cube and 1 cup water	
½ cup mixed carrots and peas	1 stalk celery, diced
½ small onion, chopped	1 small bay leaf
¼ cup tomato juice	salt and pepper
¼ cup cabbage, shredded	Worcestershire sauce, 1 teaspoon

Prepare vegetables and add to broth. Add seasonings. Boil together until vegetables are tender. Vegetables may be put through blender before adding to soup.

'49er Gold Salad
Combine ½ cup grated or shredded carrots and ½ apple and 1 tsp. raisins. Moisten with 2 tbsp. orange juice. Serve on lettuce. Use for 1 serving vegetable and 1 serving fruit.

* *From* Diabetes Mellitus; Systems of Control, *by Buris R. Boshell, M.D. Courtesy of Monoject, Division of Sherwood Medical, a Brunswick Company, St. Louis, Missouri.*

Matchstick Salad
Place a ¼ cup mound of cottage cheese on a bed of shredded let-tuce. Dip one end of crisp, tiny raw celery and carrot sticks in a bit of paprika and stick them in the cottage cheese ball, "flame" end up.

● PROBLEM: Diverticulosis and diverticulitis.

SOLUTIONS: Many physicians now treat these problems by placing the patient on a low-residue diet and gradually advancing him to a regular diet as tolerated. The following insert shows how one hospital, Mercy Hospital in Springfield, Massachusetts, plans such a diet.

LOW RESIDUE DIET

The Low Residue Diet is composed of foods that are mechanically non-irritating to the Gastro-Intestinal track. It is nutritionally adequate and is suggested for patients with diarrhea, gastro intest-inal inflammation and prior to and post intestinal surgery.

BASIC MEAL PATTERN

Breakfast:	Luncheon and Dinner
½ cup fruit or strained juice	4 OZ. strained juice or broth
½ cup cereal	3 OZ. meat or fish
1 egg	½ cup potato or substitute
1 slice toast with margarine	½ cup cooked tender vegetables
8 oz. milk	½ cup soft dessert
Beverage with milk, cream or lemon	1 slice white bread
and sugar	Margarine
	Beverage with milk, cream or lemon
	and sugar

CALORIES   1611   PRO 69 gms.   FAT 67 gms.   CHO 183 gms.

● PROBLEM: Economic restrictions.

SOLUTION: Low-budget balanced diet. Plan meals using the Basic Four Food Groups   Some of the following ways to keep food costs down are simple and practical:
  1. Buy foods according to their use. Buy small, less attractive fruits if planning to cut them up, and buy Grade B eggs for baking.
  2. Use less tender cuts of meat whenever possible.
  3. Buy large pieces of meat and plan meals around leftovers.

4. Buy "house brands" and generic brands instead of advertised brands whenever possible.
5. Buy foods in season.
6. Market at large supermarkets instead of convenience stores.
7. Use a list.
8. Plan meals around "specials."
9. Avoid compulsive buying.
10. Never shop when you are hungry.
11. Use store coupons if the product will actually be cheaper than house or generic brands. Look for double coupon days.
12. Find out if you are eligible for food stamps. If so, use them.

● PROBLEM: Loneliness.

SOLUTION: Group Dining. This is a way to ease the isolation of eating alone day after day. Most senior centers serve a daily hot meal for a nominal cost. The companionship is as important as the nutrients ingested. Perhaps occasional meals can be shared with a friend or neighbor. Churches, lodges, nondenominational clubs, and even some schools provide for group dining.

Self-Test: Do You Know Your Nutritional Facts?*

Circle T for True and F for False. Check your answers at the end of this chapter.

T	F	1.	Vitamins from natural sources are better used by the body than manmade vitamins.
T	F	2.	A balanced diet containing a variety of food can provide all the nutrition your body needs.
T	F	3.	In weight reduction, the type of fat you eat is more important than the amount.
T	F	4.	Honey is more nutritious than sugar.
T	F	5.	White bread is better for you than dark bread.
T	F	6.	Margarine has fewer calories than butter.

* Courtesy of the dietary department of Baystate Medical Center, Wesson Memorial Division, Springfield, Mass.

T	F	7.	Milk should be omitted from a reducing diet.
T	F	8.	Cooked eggs contain less cholesterol than raw eggs.
T	F	9.	Crops grown with organic fertilizers produce foods higher in nutritional value than ones grown with regular fertilizer.
T	F	10.	Everyone should take a vitamin supplement.
T	F	11.	All people should avoid eggs because of their cholesterol content.
T	F	12.	Yogurt is more nutritious than milk.
T	F	13.	Large doses of vitamin "C" protect the body from colds.
T	F	14.	Omitting salt from the diet helps in weight loss.
T	F	15.	Vitamin E supplements increase sexual potency.

A Nutritional Survey

A major part of a practical nursing program is devoted to learning about and caring for the geriatric patient. In fact, most student nurses have their initial clinical experiences with the elderly in hospitals and nursing homes. As a result, the needs of the ill aged adult take precedence in their minds over the problems of the well adult of 65 or more.

Our practical nursing students participate annually in a field trip to a nursing home or extended care facility. In 1979, we decided to have a closer look at the well adult over 65, so we visited a local Golden Age center. The students were impressed by so many elderly men and women absorbed in a wide variety of activities. Some members just dropped in each day to read their paper. We watched billiard players and observed a Weight Watchers group conduct their meeting. A lively group of square dancers, ranging up to age 85, invited us to join them and then danced rings around us. We also found out that a broad range of diversions, from crafts to a mini-course on health insurance, was available. The common interest, however, seemed to be the inexpensive noontime dinner offered. As we watched the men and women gathering in the dining room our conversation turned toward food in general and then specifically to nutritional problems of elderly people.

We devised an informal questionnaire that explored 12 categories which strongly influence the nutrition of the well adult over the age of 65. Questionnaires were distributed at random to 34 men and 34 women at the center.

Nutrition Questionnaire for the Well Adult over 65 (sample)

The following categories are included in the survey:

where meals are eaten	appetite
weekly food expenses	cooking skills
availability of markets	nutritional knowledge
shopping habits	adequacy of budget
distribution of income	nutritional problems
age range	annual income

1. Where are your meals eaten?
   _____ at home   _____ fast food restaurants
   _____ out of home   _____ communal dining

2. What is your weekly food budget?
   _____less than $12 a week   _____$15-20 a week
   _____$12-$15 a week   _____more than $20 a week

3. Is your budget satisfactory?
   ____yes   ____no____Comment:_____

4. Where are markets located?
   ____convenient walk   _____inconvenient walk
   ____convenient drive   _____must depend on others to
                                        drive
   Comment _____

5. How often do you shop?
   ____weekly   ____more than once a week
   Comment: _____

6. Where does the money go?
   ____mostly on food ____mostly on rent   ____other
   Comment: _____

7. What are carbohydrates, protein, and fat? Give an example of each.
   a. carbohydrates are useful for: _____
      an example is: _____

  b. protein is useful for: _____
       an example is: _____
  c. fat is useful for: _____
       an example is: _____

8. How is your appetite? (Circle one)
     good   fair   poor

9. How do you rate your cooking skills? (Circle one)
     good   fair   poor

10. What is your biggest nutritional problem? _____
_____

11. How old are you? (Circle one)
     65 - 70   70 - 75   80 - 85

12. What is your annual income? Please include all pensions, Social
     Security benefits, dividends, etc.
     ____$5,000 a year or less   ____$10,000 to $12,500
     ____$5,000 to $7,500   ____$12,500 to $15,000
     ____$7,500 to $10,000   ____$15,000 or more

_____

Let's look at the men's responses first.

Results of the Nutrition Questionnaire (Men)

1. *Where are your meals eaten?* Sixteen men replied that they
   ate exclusively at home. Another 16 said they ate out, but
   usually had breakfast at home. Then they ate a hot meal at a
   Lion's club, Golden Age center, or church dining facility.
   Three were thinking about signing up for Meals on Wheels.
   Two said they never ate at home—they depended on fast
   food restaurants or else they ate with their married children.

2. *What is your weekly food budget?* Nine men spent less than
   $12 a week on food. Eight spent between $12 and $15.
   Twelve spent $15 to $20, and five spent over $20.

3. *Is your budget satisfactory?* Eighteen replied that it was; fif-
   teen said it was not; and one man did not reply. Several men
   commented that they barely made ends meet; specific problems will be referred to in the answers to Question 6.

4. *Where are markets located?* Eight men said they were a convenient walk from markets, and eleven said a convenient drive. Five took a bus and ten had to depend on others to drive them or else they used Dial-a-Van.* We were surprised that only 25 percent of the men had a market they could walk to. This raised questions in our minds. For example, was this a hidden economic problem? If markets aren't nearby, then budgets escalate because of the higher prices in convenience stores and in fast food restaurants. In fact, the nutritional problem concerned us as much as the economic one. There are no fresh fruits and vegetables available in "hamburger heavens."

5. *How often do you shop?* Twenty men said they shopped weekly and 12 said they shopped several times a week. Two did not reply. Nine of the weekly shoppers said they always used a list, and most of the men said they tried to take advantage of "specials."

6. *Where does the money go?* This question must have discouraged a lot of people because half of the respondents didn't answer it. Of the 17 who did, 10 said that food claimed most of their money. Six said their income was rather evenly divided among food purchases, rent, and miscellaneous living expenses. One man wryly commented, "What money?"

7. *What are carbohydrates, protein, and fat? Give an example of each.* Nine men knew all three nutrients and gave correct examples. Twelve knew protein only and identified foods that are sources of protein. Seven men did not know the three nutrients and six men did not reply. Two men mentioned that they were on diabetic diets. Ten men felt that they ate a balanced diet but just as many did not.

8. *How is your appetite?* Sixteen men said that they had a good appetite and ten said fair. Eight did not reply. Twelve men said that they ate regular meals but five confessed to eating whenever they were hungry.

---

* *Dial-a-Van provides door to door transportation for the elderly and handicapped. People using this service reserve it 24 hours ahead of time and pay a small fee. The van takes them to medical appointments, shopping trips, or other places. The handicapped can be taken to work and back and the vans have hydraulic lifts.*

9. *How do you rate your cooking skills?* Eleven said they cooked well. Nine said they were ''fair'' cooks. Six could cook but didn't like it, and three of these added that they just did it because they had to. Three men did not know how to cook and the rest did not reply.

10. *What is the biggest nutritional problem you have?* The answers to this question fell into several classifications: transportation; money; packaging; variety; and insufficient nutritional knowledge.

    Two men claimed that distance was a problem and that they couldn't take advantage of ''specials'' when they'd like to. Four complained about packaging. They felt there was a lot of waste when a person was shopping for one. Eight men said that money was their biggest problem. Four wished they could have more variety in their diets, and two were looking for more information on nutrients. Six did not reply.

11. *How old are you?* Six men were between 65 and 70; 16 were between 70 and 75; eight were between 75 and 80; and two were between 80 and 85. Two did not reply.

12. *What is your annual income?* These were unsigned questionnaires and we asked that the respondents include all sources of income, e.g., Social Security, pensions, dividends, and so forth. The results were as follows:

    Twenty men had incomes of less than $5,000 a year. Six had incomes ranging between $5,000 and $7,500. Five were in the $7,500 to $10,000 range, and three fell into the $10,000 to $12,500 range. None had over $15,000 a year.

Results of the Nutrition Questionnaire (Women)

The responses of the 34 women were quite similar to those of the men with a few exceptions.

1. *Where are your meals eaten?* Eighteen women ate at home exclusively. Thirteen ate at home half the time and with their families or friends at other times. Three women said they never ate at home and one woman said she was nearly always at home and depended on Meals on Wheels for her food.

2. *What is your weekly food budget?* Five women spent from $12 to $15 a week; five spent less than $12; eleven spent

between $15 and $20; and 12 spent more than $20 a week.

3. *Is your budget satisfactory?* Twenty-one women said it was satisfactory and 13 said it wasn't. Some of the reasons given were that there wasn't enough money left for clothes and that Social Security was insufficient. One tongue-in-cheek comment was that there was "too much month at the end of the money." Specific problems are discussed in Question 6.

4. *Where are markets located?* Three women had markets a convenient walk from where they lived, and 14 shopped at markets a convenient drive from their homes. Seventeen said that the markets were inconveniently located and that they depended on buses, on other people driving them, and on Dial-a-Vans.

5. *How often do you shop?* Seventeen shopped weekly, 11 went more than once a week, and six did not reply. Ten said they always used a list, 16 read ads carefully and shopped the "specials," but four confessed to impulse buying.

6. *Where does the money go?* For 15, food was the most expensive item, and meat was the most costly food item. Three said they spent most of their income on rent or household expenses other than food. Sixteen did not reply.

7. *What are carbohydrates, protein, and fat? Give an example of each.* Twenty-four women knew the three nutrients and gave correct examples of each. Ten did not know them. One of these ten was diabetic and suspected that she wasn't following a very good diet.

8. *How is your appetite?* Of 17 women who said their appetites were good, 12 said they ate regular meals. One woman said her appetite was too good! Twelve said their appetites were fair, and four did not respond.

9. *How do you rate your cooking skills?* Twenty-one women said that they were good cooks. Twelve said that they were fair. Of the 12, nine said they just cooked because they had to, and two didn't like it at all. One woman said she was a poor cook.

10. *What is the biggest nutritional problem you have?* Here the answers fell into four groups: money; transportation;

loneliness; and lack of nutritional information. Twelve women said that money was their biggest problem. Five needed better transportation. Six admitted that eating too much was their problem. Three were on special diets; one of these said that finding foods without sugar was difficult, while the other two were concerned with getting enough iron in their diets. The questionnaires were anonymous, of course, and the problem of lonliness was freely expressed. One woman wrote, "I don't like to be alone when I eat and, since I am alone, I'm not interested in eating." Another said, "If I weren't alone, my eating habits would be a whole lot better than they are." Several widows claimed that they were no longer motivated to prepare meals, let alone plan and shop for them. One 80-year-old lady said that she knew her diet was not balanced, but that she had long ago lost interest in preparing meals. Only one woman out of the 34 felt that she ate a well-balanced diet.

11. *How old are you?* Twelve women were between 65 and 70; twelve were in the 70 to 75 range; and eight were between 75 and 80. Two were over 80.

12. *What is your annual income?* Seventeen women lived on $5,000 a year or less. Eleven had incomes of from $5,000 to $7,500 a year. Five lived on from $7,500 to $10,000. None were in the $10,000 to $15,000 range. Only one woman had an income over $15,000.

Similarities

Men and women paralleled each other in the following areas. About the same number ate at home or else took advantage of communal dining or fast food restaurants (Question 1). Both groups had rather similar food budgets (Question 2). Their shopping habits and expenditures were comparable (Questions 5 and 6). Men and women rated their appetites the same and they were close in age range (Questions 8 and 11).

Differences

While eight men could walk to markets (Question 4), only three women could. Not unexpectedly, a great many more women than men had better knowledge of nutrition (Question 7). Twice as

Weekly Food Budget Related to Annual Income

Income per Year	Spent on Food Each Week	Men	Women
$5,000 a year or less	less than $15	5	3
	$12 to $15	5	4
	$15 to $20	6	5
	more than $20	4	5
$5,000 to $7,500	less than $12	1	1
	$12 to $15	1	1
	$15 to $20	3	4
	more than $20	1	5
$7,500 to $10,000	less than $12	1	1
	$12 to $15	1	1
	$15 to $20	3	2
	more than $20	0	1
$10,000 to $15,000	less than $12	2	0
	$12 to $15	1	0
	$15 to $20	0	0
	more than $20	0	0
More than $15,000		0	1*

* The only respondent in this category said she spent over $20 a week.

many women as men rated themselves as good cooks (Question 9), again, no surprise. When discussing nutrition problems, men complained about waste due to packaging (Question 10). For instance, a man referred to having to buy six oranges in a pack when he wanted only one. Five went bad. The startling difference, however, surfaced in the women's questionnaires when they wrote about loneliness. This was our first glimpse into the emotional stresses of our respondents. It is also significant that the higher income groups spent less on food than the lower income groups.

Conclusions

Old people are all around us. They're there, but do we really see them? Our exploration of the nutritional practices of well adults over 65 led to many class discussions. Like most of us, the students had waited impatiently in checkout lines while elderly persons slowly counted out change, or had smiled tolerantly at old couples debating endlessly about whether to select a certain item in a store. Now the students wonder whether those fingers counting the money may be arthritic, or whether the labels are hard for those old eyes to read, or, more likely, whether the cost of the item may be the real problem. We were dismayed to learn that more than half of the respondents lived on incomes of $5,000 a year or less. Were they using food stamps, we wondered. A call to a local Council on Aging office revealed that a common problem of elderly people is that many of those who qualify for food stamps don't know it, and that those who do know it often don't know how to go about getting them. A need exists for outreach workers to find these people and help them obtain assistance.

The mention of loneliness underscored the state of most elderly women today. Not that men don't suffer from loneliness; surely they do. However, the women who wrote were of a generation where a woman's whole life centered around her husband and her children. When the husband is deceased and the children grown and gone, the quality of life can be hollow indeed.

Giving and tabulating the results of the questionnaire gave the students a better understanding of many geriatric problems.

Answers to Self-Test on page 114

(F) 1. The body uses both types of vitamins in exactly the same way.

(T) 2. A balanced diet is one which contains foods from all of the Basic 4 Food Groups.

(F) 3. All fats provide exactly the same amount of calories.

(F) 4. Honey is no more nutritious than sugar.

(F) 5. Enriched white bread provides the same nutrition as enriched dark bread.

(F) 6. Both have the same amount of calories.

(F) 7. Because milk is an excellent food, it should not be excluded from any diet. Skim milk, which omits fat, provides the same nutrition but considerably less calories than whole milk.

(F) 8. The amount of cholesterol is not changed in the cooking of eggs. It is not wise to eat raw eggs because they may carry bacteria (salmonella).

(F) 9. The nutritional value of crops grown with either kind of fertilizer is the same.

(F) 10. Vitamin supplements are unnecessary if basic four foods are included in the daily diet.
(F) 11. Most people do not have to restrict eating eggs if their body uses cholesterol properly.
(F) 12. Plain yogurt provides the same nutrition as whole milk from which it is made.
(F) 13. It has not been definitely proven that Vitamin "C" prevents the common cold.
(F) 14. Omitting salt *may* help weight loss, but your doctor should be consulted before undertaking any type of diet.
(F) 15. It has not been proven that Vitamin E increases sexual potency.

ACTIVITIES

1. Develop a brief nutrition questionnaire for the single adult over the age of 65.
2. Select 12 charts of patients at random. How many have a recorded height and weight on admission?
3. Read six charts of patients who are NPO or on IVs. When did they have their last solid food?
4. Find out if any hospital in your area does a nutritional assessment test. Describe it.

PART II

Nursing Procedures and Measures

Introduction

An elderly man was a patient in a prestigious medical center. A dietitian noted his food allergies and preferences; his x-rays and laboratory tests were competently handled; and his medications and vital signs were managed by a skilled team. The patient had been given several laxatives and enemas in preparation for x-ray exams, and as a result, he became very weak. In fact, he was unable to stand without assistance. Yet, in all this time, he had not been given a bath of any kind. Clearly a nursing omission. Oh, a *nurse* didn't have to bathe him. Perhaps a nursing assistant could have done that. But somewhere along the line a nurse should have supervised better personal care.

Sometimes it seems that the fragmentation of nursing actually begins in the classroom as a covert lesson students learn along with anatomy, biology, pharmacology, and nutrition. Nursing programs require a dizzying array of courses. However, patients aren't jigsaw puzzles. Students can't memorize symptoms, laboratory reports, medications, and diet therapy, and then group them all together and come up with a complete picture of a patient. Instructors have the responsibility of insisting that the students who look at a patient see an individual. The ideal place to do this is in the fundamentals procedure laboratory.

It's very difficult for a healthy young student nurse to appreciate the impact of hospitalization and its disruptive effect on people. They may listen to lectures on the dependent patient and study assignments on the "activities of daily living." But it's not until they match lectures to assignments in the procedure laboratory and actually give each other bedside care that they gain some insight into the meaning of dependency.

There has been a trend among teachers of nursing to rely on visual aids because of the ever-increasing amount of material that has to be taught in a steadily shrinking period of time. Granted, there isn't a procedure that hasn't been taped or filmed to perfection. The quality available is superb. Instructors like these aids because it helps them introduce new material or reinforce what has been taught. Students like them for the same reasons and, in addition, they can review at their own pace. Everybody likes the AVs. They are excellent supplements to classroom teaching. But that's all they are. Supplements. They are not designed to replace the practice in the procedure laboratory. There is no film on the bed bath quite as dramatic in its effect as actually feeling a cold washcloth on your back!

As a fundamentals instructor, I have found that the procedure laboratory offers an opportunity for many learning situations besides acquiring and perfecting skills. Techniques can be taught and must be practiced. This is part of the science of nursing. But what about empathy, rapport, and understanding? These qualities belong to the art of nursing and it is in this area that the student is largely self-taught. The procedure laboratory affords a setting in which to become introspective and to perceive the evolution of attitudes and feelings.

For example, Barbara, a student who had been the "patient" in a laboratory exercise on the bed bath, voiced her negative feelings when told to prepare for this procedure. She confessed to feeling very nervous because she didn't like the idea of a stranger touching her. However, since her "nurse" drew the curtains and was careful to drape her with a bath blanket, she never felt exposed. Barbara learned proper draping and how to give a bed bath. Equally important, she understood the reason behind a patient's anxiety about the procedure.

Anne, another student, agreed that draping was important, but she pointed out that there is also a sudden loss of dignity when a stranger has control over your body. She suggested that the nurse might try to relax her patient with conversation. "Of course, you have to be careful of what you say because it's possible to embarrass people when you notice their scars, rashes, or bruises—but what a good chance for making observations and getting acquainted with your patient."

"To think that we call going to the bathroom a privilege!" exclaimed Claire, a student who tried sitting on a bedpan before her "nurse" bathed her. "I wouldn't want to stay on *that* too long." Claire couldn't wait to get the bath over with. The water was either too hot or too cold. She felt sticky because Eve, her "nurse," didn't rinse her thoroughly. "I was embarrassed being bathed by a classmate, but I'm glad we did this because I had a chance to be in the patient's shoes."

Eve noted that this experience was important for empathy. "And I'll be more organized next time. I'll remember to change the water when it cools off, and I'll try not to forget to have a clean 'johnnie' on hand."

Ben, a relaxed, confident student, couldn't wait to tell about his participation in a laboratory exercise on feeding. "It was awful not being able to lift a spoon or a glass. The food came at me too fast and I was very self-conscious about how much I was swallowing and chewing. I was afraid of juice dripping down my neck and crumbs kept falling out of my mouth. I couldn't enjoy anything. To make matters worse, my 'nurse' never used my napkin. Either she didn't think I spilled enough or she just didn't see it. Finally I had to tell her. But suppose I couldn't?"

Erik, the other man in the class, agreed that it's important to remember things like not going too fast or too slow. "I just wished my 'nurse' had talked to me," he said, "but she just stood there watching my mouth and spooning it in. I had the feeling it was just a chore she had to do and that made me uncomfortable."

The discussion turned to oral care. "I remember reading the chapter before we practiced this," Claire said smiling. "I thought, 'this is going to be easy.' But I forgot how sensitive the mouth is. My 'nurse' couldn't seem to get the brush into the right places. She brushed too hard and hurt my gums. The worst of it was having to spit into that little basin. Now *that* was embarrassing.''

Ben said, ''The toothbrush was never at the right angle. Toothpaste was everywhere. All over my chin, on my mouth—even up my nose. Now I understand what it's like to be on the receiving end. I knew right from the beginning I wasn't going to like this. I'm self-conscious about my teeth and I didn't like the idea of someone else deciding when they were clean.''

Admittedly, oral care, feeding, and the bed bath are not as technically demanding as dressings, blood pressures, or catheterizations. Instructors have to set priorities and the more complex procedures require more time. But every effort should be made to include the basic methods of personal care. They are important components of bedside nursing and provide meaningful patient contact in the clinical area. Carrying out these procedures offer valuable opportunities to assess needs.

The charge of insensitive treatment has been leveled against many health care facilities. One nursing home made news recently when the staff took a close look at themselves and decided upon a novel inservice experience. Everyone from the administrator to the custodian participated, and they spent time in restraints, in wheelchairs, and in bed. Ears were stuffed with cotton pledgets to impair hearing, and, if glasses were worn, they were smudged with Vaseline to simulate blurry vision. No one knew when it would be his turn at being the ''patient.'' And it didn't matter whether the participant was conducting a meeting or was headed for the bathroom! The person selected was abruptly placed in a wheelchair and assumed the role of ''patient'' for the day. The immediate result of the innovative program was a heightened awareness of the patient's basic needs.

General Rules for Procedures

1. Verify the order before beginning *any* procedure by checking either the chart or the kardex.
2. Identify the patient, introduce yourself, and explain the procedure.

3. Assemble the necessary equipment carefully to avoid running out of the room at the last minute. Remember containers for wastes (soiled dressings), basins for irrigating solutions, clean "johnnies" for bed baths, and so on.

4. Use curtains, screens, and bath blankets for draping to insure privacy.

5. Adapt the procedure to the individual. If a confused, incontinent patient can't stay in Sims' position for an enema, give it to him on a bedpan. Wear gloves!

6. Wash your hands before and after procedures. Wash the patient's hands whenever necessary.

7. Remember aftercare of patients following procedures, whenever necessary, and remember to remove and/or replace used equipment.

8. Chart what was done, when it was done, the results, your observations, and the patient's reaction when appropriate.

9. Remember that a patient has a right to refuse a procedure. Simply report this to the appropriate person and document the refusal.

A NOTE ON HANDWASHING: * Conscientious aseptic technique is the best way to check the insidious spread of nosocomial infections. The times to wash your hands include: when hands look soiled; before and after direct patient contact, especially of the face and mouth; after toileting; after blowing or wiping your nose; upon leaving an isolation area or handling articles from one; after handling dressings, specimens, catheters, and bedpans; before eating; and before leaving the health care facility.

This is the standard hand-washing procedure:

1. Wet your hands with warm running water.
2. Lather well with soap.
3. Scrub for at least 15 seconds.
4. Direct your hands downward into the sink. This keeps contaminated water from running onto your forearms.
5. If necessary, clean under your nails.
6. Dry your hands with a paper towel.
7. Turn off the faucet with a towel. Remember, those germs you washed away are now all over the sink.

* From "Are You Fudging on Hand-Washing Routines?" by Joan Breitung, RN Magazine, *June, 1977.*

Functional Losses Associated with Age — Capsulized for Quick Reference

Heart: This may decrease in size but more frequently increases in size as a consequence of congestive heart failure. Cardiac output decreases and there is less ability of the heart to respond to stressful situations such as infections.

Kidney: There is a definite decrease of functioning nephrons. There is a substantial decrease in renal blood flow and glomerulo filtration rate.

Liver: Here also, there is a definite decrease in size and hepatic capacity with advanced age. Enzyme function usually remains adequate *except* in the area of drug metabolism.

Lungs: Lung composition decreases in elastic potential and shows an increase in collagen and rigidity. The dimensions of the thoracic cage increase with hyperinflation of the lung tissue. There is also a decrease in ciliary movement.

Neurons: There is a decided decrease in brain weight and number of neurons. There is a decrease in the conduction velocity of peripheral nerves.

Endocrine: Decrease in hormonal secretions, especially gonadal steroids. Diminished function of pancreas is determined by a lowering of the insulin secreted from the beta cells and released into the blood stream. Also, blood glucose levels require a longer period of time to return to normal after heavy glucose intake (in the elderly).

Blood Vessels: There is a fraying of elastic fibers with calcification. An increase in the collagen content and thickness of the vessel walls with a decrease in resiliency results. The resulting atherosclerosis leads to a narrowing in blood vessels contributing to diminished blood flow. If the atherosclerosis is in the coronary arteries, (and it usually is) cardiac output is reduced.

Eye: There is loss of corneal endothelial cells with decreased sensitivity. The anterior chamber becomes shallow. The iris loses pigment and the pupil becomes gradually smaller. The lens becomes more opaque.

Ear: Presbycusis, mild progressive bilateral hearing loss, does not cause deafness in itself, but it *is* irreversible.

Immunity: Immunologic tolerance for self-preservation decreases.

8

The Integumentary System

Objectives

After completing this chapter, the student should be able to:
- describe the purposes of the skin
- explain what causes changes in the skin of the aged
- carry out procedures for rubs and the various types of baths
- give care for decubitus ulcers
- care for the hair, nails, and feet of patients
- use the following words correctly

Vocabulary

The following words relate to the material in this chapter. Look up the ones you do not know or are not sure of.

axilla	Fowler's position	perineal area
callus	incontinence	podiatrist
coccyx	keratosis	sacrum
decubitus ulcer	labia	sebum
epithelial	pendulous	subcutaneous

Anatomy Review

The skin is one of the body's largest organs.

Structures

Epidermis.   This outer layer of the skin is continually being shed and replaced. It has nerve endings but no blood vessels.

Dermis.   The dermis lies beneath the epidermis. It contains blood vessels, nerve endings, hair follicles, sebaceous glands, and sweat glands.

Hair Follicles.   These are small sacs that contain the hair roots.

Nails.   Nails are made of keratin, a tough protein. They protect the ends of the fingers and toes.

Sebaceous Glands. These secrete an oily substance called sebum.

Sweat Glands.   These secrete sweat.

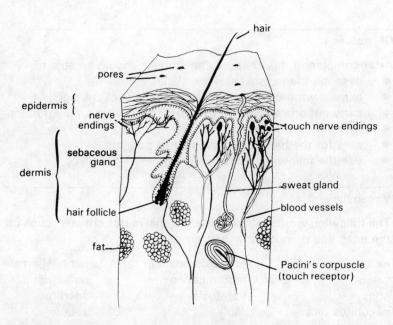

Schematic drawing of a section of the skin

Functions Include
  heat regulation
  acting as a protective barrier

The sweat glands, twisted tubules buried in the dermis, function to eliminate water and control heat loss from the body. The skin is a protective barrier because it acts as a shield against the invasion of the body by microorganisms.

Age-Related Changes

1. *Wrinkles.* These signal advancing years and they are caused by decreased subcutaneous fat and elastic fibers.
2. *Dry Skin.* The skin becomes dry as the production of sebum, nature's lubricant, by the sebaceous glands lessens.
3. *Pruritus.* The maddening itch of pruritus that accompanies dryness is a common complaint of the elderly patient. (*NOTE:* symptoms of disease and drug reactions can also cause pruritus.)
4. *Keratoses.* These benign scaly growths often found on the face and head, are frequently seen in the elderly.
5. *Brittle Nails.* Fingernails and toenails become ridged and brittle. They should be kept short and smooth. If the nurse isn't able to care for the toenails of the elderly patient safely, a podiatrist should be consulted.
6. *Dry Hair.* The hair of the elderly is generally thin because of reduction of the activity of the follicles. Dryness again may be a problem because of scant sebum production.
7. *Decubitus Ulcers (Bedsores).* These often occur on patients confined to bed for long periods of time, as many elderly patients are. Although this is not an age-related phenomenon, it is a factor in caring for aged patients.

Nursing Procedures

The Bed Bath
In health care facilities, much "AM care" time is devoted to giving bed baths. Done correctly, they leave the patient comfortable, relaxed, and refreshed in body and spirit.

Bathtime is an excellent time to assess a patient. The nurse can observe the skin for color, texture, rashes, or scars. Equally important is that the bath giver has an opportunity to know the patient.

There's a disadvantage, though. The cleansing bed bath, given by someone else, offers only passive exercise. So the sooner the patient is able to bathe himself, the sooner he benefits from active exercise and a sense of independence.

Most baths are given in the morning after breakfast. But all baths don't have to be done then. The nurse's schedule should be flexible enough to accommodate a patient who's just dozed off after a sleepless night.

Purposes
to bathe patients who can't get out of bed
to identify skin abnormalities

Equipment

bath blanket	face towel	soap
basin	gown	deodorant
bath towel	wash cloth	lotion
		powder

Sequence

1. identify patient; introduce self; explain procedure
2. see that room temperature is comfortable
3. insure privacy with screens, curtains, or draping
4. check dressings (change as indicated)
5. replace top sheet and spread with the bath blanket
6. remove gown, eyeglasses, wristwatch, and so on
7. fill basin ¾ full of water 110°F (use bath thermometer)
8. place patient in low Fowler's position, near to the side of the bed
9. lay small hand towel on top of bath blanket over chest
10. ask if soap is used on face; wet cloth, wring out
11. make a mitt out of cloth by clasping the corners between thumb and fingers (instuctor illustrates)
12. wash and rinse face, neck, ears; blot dry

13. uncover *far* arm: wash and rinse, using long, smooth strokes; dry arm and axilla; apply deodorant
14. repeat with near arm
15. let patient place hands in basin if possible; wash, rinse, dry hands; clean nails
16. place bath towel over chest; fold bath blanket to waist; wash, rinse, and dry; observe for excoriations in skin folds under pendulous breasts of obese females; treat as per hospital policy
17. wash *far* leg using long, smooth strokes; if possible, place basin on the bed, flex patient's knee, cup your hand to support heel and lower foot into basin (instructor illustrates); wash, rinse and dry; repeat for other leg; care for toenails as per institution's policy
18. change bath water
19. turn patient and wash and rinse back; back rub may be given at this time or after bath is completed
20. Place patient again in low Fowler's position; place equipment near patient; tell him to complete personal bath (genital area) if he is able,or complete bath for helpless patient

NOTES: When giving perineal care to the incontinent, uncircumsized male patient, retract the foreskin (prepuce) while washing the penis in order to remove secretions that can cause odor and irritation. When genital hygiene is complete, draw foreskin back over the penis. Turn patient on his side, lift buttock, wash anal area, rinse and dry.

The female patient benefits from being placed on a bedpan and having a pitcher of warm water poured over the vulva. The labia must be separated carefully to give genital hygiene to the female patient.

Improper draping and screening of patients violates not only their dignity but also their rights.

The Tub Bath

Immersing hands or feet in a basin of water adds considerably to the enjoyment of the bath. When a person is able to get into a tub of warm water and soak, the bath becomes a doubly pleasurable experience.

The nurse must take precautions against skids and falls (for the nurse as well as the patient!). A nonskid tub mat is as important as a dry floor. The door is not locked even for the alert, reliable self-care patient. Plan to check on the patient within five minutes. Point out the emergency call light to patient.

Purpose
to bathe the patient in a bathtub safely and effectively.

Equipment
bath blanket   soap   bath mat
two bath towels   tub mat (or towel)   chair
wash cloth

Sequence
1. identify patient; introduce self; explain procedure
2. inspect tub to be sure it is clean; fill half full of water 110°F
3. have patient test water before getting into tub
4. place mat or towel in tub
5. caution patient to use handrail; assist as needed
6. assist with bath or leave patient alone as situation indicates
7. indicate call signal to patient; return in five minutes; wash back; observe skin for abnormalities
8. assist patient out of tub, dry and help dress as necessary
9. clean tub and leave it presentable for next patient

The Back Rub
Giving a good back rub is as satisfying for the nurse as getting a back rub is for the patient. The actual "laying on of hands" reinforces the nursing role of comforter. At the end of the back rub, the patient should feel comfortable, relaxed, and cared for.

If the patient can tolerate it, he should lie on his abdomen. Otherwise, the side-lying position is used. Beginning at the base of the spine, the nurse uses long, smooth strokes that travel up the back, part at the base of the neck, and then glide downward so the hands meet at the coccyx.

Purposes

to relieve tension.

to promote circulation of the skin and help prevent decubitus ulcers.

Equipment

towel   lotion   powder   gown

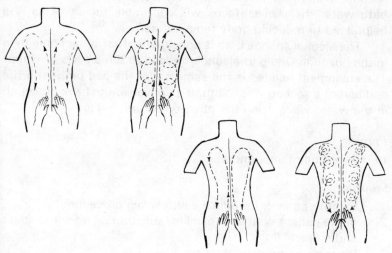

The back rub. Arrows indicate directions in which hands move. Circles indicate areas to massage. Sacral area requires extra massage.

Sequence

1. identify patient; introduce self; explain procedure
2. screen patient
3. open back of gown
4. pour small amount of lotion into palm of hand to take chill off lotion; rub hands together
5. place hands together, palms down on coccyx
6. slide hands up backbone, exerting pressure
7. separate hands at neck; slide hands down back

8. inspect skin for reddened areas
9. massage coccyx area to stimulate circulation
10. continue back rub for from three to five minutes
11. blot dry with towel
12. powder sparingly, if desired; remove gown and put fresh gown on patient

Alcohol Sponge Bath
Alcohol evaporates faster than water, so if alcohol is added to bath water the skin surfaces will cool more rapidly. This is a helpful aid to reducing body temperature.

The alcohol sponge bath is done more often in the home than in the hospital. One part alcohol is added to three parts of water. The equipment needed is the same as for the bed bath with the addition of a second washcloth. It's convenient to have one cloth in the water while using the other on an arm or leg.

Purpose
to reduce body temperature

Sequence
1. identify patient; introduce self; explain procedure
2. drape patient with bath blanket, substituting it for top sheet and spread
3. leave gown on patient
4. wash left arm and axilla; dry
5. wash left leg; dry
6. wash right leg; dry
7. wash right arm and axilla; dry
8. wash and dry back

The chest and abdomen are omitted. A cold cloth (or icebag) on the forehead relieves the headache that accompanies fever. A hot water bottle at the feet is a comfort measure to prevent chilling.

The patient is draped so that only the part of the body being bathed is exposed. The entire procedure takes about 20 minutes. The patient's temperature should be taken before and after the procedure.

The Sitz Bath

There are special tubs designed so that patients sit in them and only the rectal, buttock, and perineal areas are bathed. There are also portable basins that may be used to administer sitz baths in the home and in the hospital.

A sitz bath is usually prescribed by a physician to relieve pain and encourage wound healing when someone has had rectal surgery. Occasionally they're ordered to relieve urine retention. Warm water 110°F to 115°F produces maximum effects within 15 minutes.

Purposes
to relieve rectal pain and promote healing
to recognize untoward effects

Equipment
towel or air ring for tub	bath mat	chair
towel for drying patient	bath blanket	

Sequence
1. identify patient; introduce self; explain procedure
2. draw bath for patient; test temperature of water; place towel or air ring in tub
3. drape bath blanket around patient's shoulders
4. maintain proper body alignment while patient is sitting in tub
5. aftercare, dressing change as per physician's order

A sitz tub is better than a regular bathtub because there is more concentration of heated water on the anal-pelvic region. The nurse should observe carefully for patient's weakness, color change, or dizziness while soak is being given.

Decubitus Ulcers

People who are confined to bed for long periods of time are especially prone to the skin breakdown commonly called bedsores. These ulcers occur over the bony prominences of the body, i.e., sacrum, heel, and tops of hips (iliac crests), although any area of the body where there is prolonged pressure can be subject to decubiti. The ulcers form because there is interference with the circulation that nourishes the skin. Ulceration is the result of this interference.

Purposes of Decubitus Ulcer Care
to recognize the beginning decubitus ulcer
to prevent the formation of decubiti
to care for the patient with decubiti

Prevention
Decubitus ulcers can be prevented if the following steps are taken:
1. keep the skin meticulously clean and dry
2. change the patient's position at least every two hours
3. keep the sheets dry and wrinkle free
4. massage the pressure areas
5. encourage good nutrition and adequate fluid intake
6. inspect bony prominences frequently; pale mottled skin or a

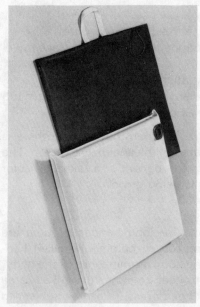

The flotation pad changes the pressure points and aids in preventing decubitus ulcers.

reddened area may be the beginning of a decubitus ulcer; in a short period of time, the reddened area becomes irritated, the skin sloughs off, and a bedsore is in full bloom.

Caring for Decubitus Ulcers
There are many effective ways to care for these ulcers. Some devices used are:

Air Mattresses. These distribute the pressure of the body so no one area of the body is subjected to pressure for a long period of time.

Sheepskins. These allow air circulation and keep the skin dry.

Heel and Elbow Protectors. These prevent pressure and allow circulation of air.

Flotation Units. These are pads or water beds.

NOTE: Heel and elbow protectors must be taken off daily at bath time. After the patient's skin is washed and dried, lotion is applied, and the protectors are replaced.

While the best policy is to prevent decubitus ulcers from occurring in the first place, the time eventually comes when the nurse has to face the problem. There have been many remedies: egg whites and sugar, karaya powder, peroxide irrigations, heat lamps, and oxygen, to mention but a few. Most health care facilities have standard policies for the treatment of decubiti. However, no treatment will meet with success unless there is continuity of care on each shift. At the very least, the patient must be kept clean and dry, turned at regular intervals, and adequately hydrated.

Care of the Hair
Keeping the patient's hair neatly and attractively arranged is an important part of daily patient care. Depending on the patient's condition, the nurse may comb the hair either while the patient is in bed or after the bath when the patient is sitting up in a chair. It is usually easier to do this procedure when the patient is in a chair.

Purposes
to keep hair and scalp clean and healthy
to improve the patient's appearance
to encourage a feeling of well-being through grooming

Equipment

comb
towel
brush
hairpins or rubber bands (if patient is female)

Sequence
1. place towel over the patient's shoulders
2. brush or comb small sections of hair at a time, starting at the *ends* of the hair and working upwards
3. alcohol may be applied to snarls of oily hair; Vaseline may be used on the snarls of dry hair
4. observe the scalp for lesions and the hair for parasites (lice, nits)
5. long hair may be braided and secured with elastics

NOTE: Hair is never cut by a nurse except in emergency situations.

Shampoo in Bed

Generally, a physician's order is needed to give a patient confined to bed a shampoo. If the patient can tolerate it, i.e., isn't too weak, tired, or running a fever, the shampoo is refreshing and aids considerably in improving spirits as well as appearance.

Some hospital beds are constructed so that the headboard lifts off. In this case, a nurse can stand at the head of the bed holding a basin to catch the water another nurse pours over the patient's head. An alternative to a bed shampoo might be to get the patient on a stretcher and into the utility room where a shampoo may be given over a sink or hopper.

Equipment

bath towels	pail or basin for	rubber or plastic
2 pitchers	catching waste	sheeting
liquid shampoo	water	waterproof protective pads

Sequence
1. move patient as close to edge of bed as possible
2. protect bedding by using rubber or plastic sheeting under heat and shoulders of patient; cover this sheeting with towels or a bath blanket
3. direct the end of the sheeting into a pail or basin on a footstool to form a kind of trough; water will be poured over the head and should run down the trough into the pail
4. lather the hair and scalp, then rub thoroughly; rinse; repeat as necessary
5. dry hair with a towel

   NOTE: The ambulatory patient may comfortably be shampooed at the bathroom sink or, in some cases, if the sink is too high, over the toilet. The nurse should observe the patient carefully for signs of weakness. If this occurs, the shampoo is stopped and the patient is returned to bed.

Hair Care for the Black Patient
The liquid shampoo generally used on patients may not be suitable for the naturally dry, coarse, very curly hair of the black patient. The nurse should determine if there are any allergies to oil or alcohol. Then, with the patient's and physician's permission, a mixture of one part alcohol to four parts mineral oil can be massaged into the scalp and hair, and toweled off. A wide-toothed afro comb can then be used to arrange the hair suitably.

Care of Nails
Included in daily hygiene is care of the fingernails and toenails. Fingernails may be cleaned with an orangewood stick after the bath. Rough or jagged nails should be smoothed with an emery board.

   The toenails (especially those of the elderly patient), are more difficult to care for. They may be thickened and brittle and hard to cut. If, after giving the patient a thorough footsoak and using an emery board to smooth the toenails, the nurse finds that the elderly patient needs more attention than the nurse can give, a podiatrist should be sent for. Bandage scissors are unsuitable and toenail clippers are risky to use on an elderly patient, and the podiatrist has the special instruments and skill with which to solve the problem.)

The Foot Soak

After the bed bath has been given, if the patient's condition permits him to be out of bed he should be allowed to sit in a chair and soak his feet. A towel or newspaper is spread on the floor under the basin of warm water. The patient can soak his feet while the nurse makes the bed. Then the feet are thoroughly dried, lotion is applied, and socks or slippers are put on. This makes up in a small way for not being able to take a shower or tub bath!

DIABETIC PRECAUTIONS: Poor circulation is a problem among diabetics and foot care is part of patient teaching if the nurse is caring for a diabetic patient. Meticulous skin care is mandatory and it should consist of washing, drying between each toe and keeping the toenails trimmed straight across. Footwear must be scrupulously clean. Above all, the diabetic must avoid treating corns, calluses, and so on, with any home remedies. The only one competent to care for these foot problems is a podiatrist.

REVIEW

A. Multiple Choice (Select the Best Answer)

1. The outer layer of the skin is called
   a. follicle
   b. tubule
   c. epidermis
   d. sebum
2. The bed bath is an excellent time to
   a. explain the hospital routine
   b. assess skin abnomalities
   c. lower body temperature
   d. use cold water for rinsing
3. Improper draping and screening
   a. irritates the doctor
   b. confuses the patient
   c. violates the patient's rights
   d. lowers the nurse's performance evaluation

4. When administering a back rub the nurse should
   a. verify the physician's order with the supervisor
   b. pour a small amount of lotion into her hands to take the chill off the lotion
   c. follow the back rub with plenty of powder
   d. put the patient in Sims' position
5. The alcohol sponge bath is given to
   a. reduce body temperature
   b. relieve tension
   c. assess skin abnormalities
   d. enable the nurse to complete the nursing care plan

B. Matching Test (Match Column 1 with column 2)

Column 1

a. the bed bath
b. rectal surgery, ordered post-op
c. bedsore
d. permits circulation of air to skin
e. stimulates circulation and relieves tension

Column 2

_____6. sitz bath
_____7. decubitus ulcer
_____8. sheepskin
_____9. backrub
_____10. passive exercise

C. Briefly Answer the Following Questions

1. In what ways might shampooing and grooming the hair of the black patient differ from caring for the hair of a white patient?
2. What are some common useful means of preventing decubitus ulcers?
3. How does the skin of an elderly patient differ from that of a young adult?
4. What are the precautions the nurse can teach to a diabetic patient concerning foot care?
5. Explain why the hair of the elderly patient is usually thin.

9

The Respiratory System

Objectives

After completing this chapter, the student should be able to:

- understand more clearly the structure and function of the lungs and related organs
- explain what causes changes in the respiratory system of the aged
- carry out postural drainage, inhalations, specimen collection, oxygen therapy, oral suctioning, and tracheostomy suctioning procedures
- help patients do breathing exercises
- use the following words correctly

Vocabulary

The following words relate to the material in this chapter. Look up the ones you do not know or are not sure of.

allergen	dyspnea	mucous
aspirate	emesis	mucus
bronchodilator	expectorant	nebulizer
bronchiectasis	flowmeter	osteoporosis
cyanosis	kyphosis	uvula

Anatomy Review

Breathing is essential to life. It is so important that we call it vital. That is why timing respirations is called taking a vital sign.

Functions

The word "respiration" means an exchange of gases between an organism and the environment in which it lives. The respiratory system involves internal and external respiration.

Internal Respiration. This type of respiration takes place in the *cells.* Through a series of complex changes, the food we ingest is oxidized (burned). Oxygen is used to free the energy from our food. Some of this energy is used to stabilize body temperature and some of it is used directly by muscle cells.

External Respiration. Oxygen is delivered to the cells of the body by way of the bloodstream. Carbon dioxide, a waste product, is carried away by the same means. The actual process works this way: a person inhales; air enters alveoli, which are air sacs in the lungs; oxygen from that air passes through membranes that line the sacs and joins the red blood cells. The bloodstream carries oxygen along to the heart, which then distributes it to the rest of the body by means of its ceaseless pumping action. At the same time, carbon dioxide leaves the blood and gets collected briefly in the alveolar sacs until the person exhales.

Structures

Lungs. Our lungs are paired, triangular organs located in the thoracic cavity. The tip of the triangle is called the apex. The bottom is called the base. The lungs "stand" on the diaphragm, the muscle that serves as a partition between the thoracic cavity and the abdominal cavity. The right lung has three lobes (sections) and the left has two.

Lungs are spongy and are enclosed in a membrane called pleura. This membrane is double because it not only covers the lungs but also lines the thoracic cavity. It secretes a fluid which prevents friction between the two layers.

Alveolus.   An alveolus is an air sac enclosed in a membrane richly supplied with capillaries.

Bronchiole.   A stem-like entrance to the alveolus. It branches to form larger bronchi.

Bronchus.   A large tubular structure; extends to bronchioles.

Trachea. The trachea channels air to the thorax. It is framed with cartilage rings.

Diaphragm.   This is the floor of thoracic cavity. It curves upward. It contracts with each inspiration.

Intercostals.   The external muscles between ribs. They raise the ribs and enlarge the thorax upon inspiration.

Ribs.   The 12 pairs of ribs form a bony cage which protects lungs and heart.

This system is best visualized as a series of tunnels. We inhale air through the nose, which is lined with a warm, moist, mucous membrane that warms and moistens the air we breathe in.

The air continues down the pharynx, past the larynx (voicebox), and into the trachea. The trachea is the trunk of what

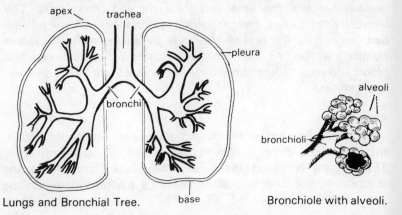

Lungs and Bronchial Tree.   Bronchiole with alveoli.

we refer to as the bronchial tree. The trachea then branches out to a right and left bronchus. "Twigs" of these bronchi are bronchioles, minute tunnels in a system of tunnels that end in microscopic air sacs called alveoli. Alveoli are surrounded by a rich network of capillaries. A comparison might be a blossom (the alveoli) on a stem (the bronchiole). It is in the alveoli that the exchange of gases takes place. The air we breathe in has a higher concentration of oxygen than does the blood in the capillaries surrounding the alveoli. Therefore, the oxygen passes from the alveoli to the capillaries. The reverse is true of carbon dioxide. The carbon dioxide in the capillaries passes into the alveoli to be exhaled.

Age-Related Changes and Conditions

The aging process brings about changes in the skeletal and muscular systems that can adversely affect the respiratory system. These include:

1. The rib cage becomes rigid as the costal cartilages calcify.
2. Osteoporosis and kyphosis (humpback) cause a stooped posture which decreases the ability of the chest to expand with each inspiration.
3. The abdominal muscles usually become weaker and lack tone, and then the diaphragm, an important organ of respiration, is affected.
4. The lungs lose some of their elasticity. Bronchioles and alveoli enlarge and decrease in number; their walls become thin and less elastic.
5. Arteriosclerosis prevents the forceful circulation of the blood; thus it is harder to circulate blood through the lungs.

All of these changes contribute to poor exchange of oxygen and carbon dioxide in the lungs and make respiratory diseases more serious in the elderly adult. However, despite this, older people are usually able to breathe quite normally.

Chronic obstructive pulmonary disease (COPD) occurs more frequently in the older age group. Emphysema, chronic bronchitis, and asthma are examples of this unfortunate situation.

Emphysema

In this condition the alveoli are overdistended and filled with air. This distends the lungs and the heart must work increasingly harder to push blood through the lungs.

Causes: smoking; exposure to pollutants in air; chronic asthma

Symptoms: expectoration of thick sputum, especially in the morning; shortness of breath; wheezing; coughing; large "barrel" chest

Treatment: bronchodilators to relieve bronchospasm; postural drainage; antibiotics to combat infection; use of nebulizers to help liquefy secretions; breathing exercise; intermittent positive pressure breathing therapy

The patient who has emphysema needs tremendous emotional support. His disease is progressive and exhausting. He leans forward in a chair with his shoulders hunched, neck muscles contracted, and lips pursed as he tries to conserve the strength and effort that make breathing, which is normally an involuntary function, very difficult. Eating is exhausting and he has little appetite. Weight loss is inevitable. He soon becomes an invalid and death usually occurs as a result of secondary infection or enlargement of the right ventricle of the heart. His heart fails because his lungs cease to function.

Chronic Bronchitis

This condition frequently progresses to emphysema or bronchiectasis.

Causes: irritants (including cigarettes); infections; hereditary factors.

Symptoms: coughing and expectoration of profuse, thick mucous secretions, especially early in the morning; dyspnea upon exertion; cyanotic lips; abdominal breathing

Treatment: bronchodilators; postural drainage; chest physical therapy (percussion, vibration); increased fluid intake; prevention of infection

Nursing care is similar to that for emphysema, including the following recommendations:

attention to nutrition

increased fluid intake (helps liquefy secretions)

rest, relaxation (exercises in selected cases as per physician's order)

use of a humidifier

avoidance of exposure to irritants in the atmosphere

influenza immunization (if physician orders it)

good oral hygiene (to reduce multiplication of disease producing microorganisms)

Asthma

Causes: chemical reactions in the body; emotional reactions; food; irritants in the atmosphere

Symptoms: wheezing; dyspnea; cyanosis

Treatment: bronchodilators; expectorants; corticosteroids; intermittent positive pressure breathing (IPPB); careful use of sedatives; avoidance of precipitating factors, e.g., stress, exposure to allergens

Status Asthmaticus

This is a serious episode of asthma that doesn't seem to respond to the usual treatments. Intensive respiratory treatment by the physician and the respiratory therapy staff is needed. This is an emergency situation.

Lung Cancer

This disease is more often seen in middle-aged persons than in geriatric patients. However, if surgery is indicated for an elderly patient with lung cancer, the usual surgical risks are involved. Should chemotherapy be the treatment of choice, lower doses are prescribed than for a middle-aged patient.

Since tumors grow more slowly in the aged, the cause of mortality is usually other than cancer.

Nursing Measures and Procedures

Postural Drainage

Postural drainage is achieved by positioning a patient so that secretions can drain from the respiratory tract. The head and chest should be lower than the hips. This way the force of gravity helps drain secretions from the smaller bronchi into the trachea, where they are removed either by coughing or by suctioning.

Vibration and percussion may be ordered along with postural drainage to help free the mucus. Vibration consists of applying firm pressure with the fingers and then moving them (as in a tremor) to the chest to help free mucus. Percussion is the rhythmic tapping of the chest for the same purpose. These techniques are used by respiratory therapists as well as by nurses.

Effective postural drainage is done before meals and at bedtime. The positions can be modified for elderly patients who are unable to assume the more basic position of postural drainage. Aftercare includes collection of a specimen if ordered and proper disposal of the sputum, tissues, paper bag, and so on, as well as thorough oral hygiene for the patient. Documentation should include color, amount, and consistency of sputum, and tolerance of the procedure.

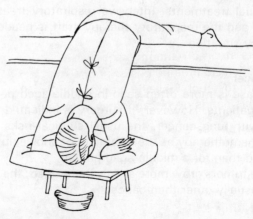

Position for Postural Drainage.

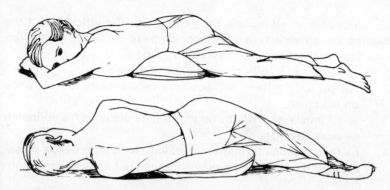

Positions in bed for postural drainage. Pillows are used to elevate the hips and the lower part of the abdomen.

Breathing Exercises

Breathing, the act of inhaling and exhaling, and coughing, the clearing of the air passages, are two acts we generally take for granted. However, physical changes in the aged may make either or both actions difficult and ineffective. If an elderly person has COPD, breathing exercises will be prescribed. The problem is that these patients tend to breathe rapidly and shallowly from the upper chest. They need to be taught how to breathe so as to empty the lungs, place less strain on the abdominal muscles, and promote relaxation. A good time to do this is right after the patient has engaged in postural drainage. For example:

1. place the patient in a sitting position with his trunk slightly forward, his feet on the floor, and his knees and hips flexed to take strain off abdominal muscles
2. tell patient to breathe in slowly and deeply through the nose
3. tell him to cough while he breathes out and to exert pressure with his hands on his abdomen with each cough

Another simple exercise for any elderly person to do to improve his breathing efficiency is the following:

1. breathe through the nose in any position of comfort (sitting, standing, lying down)
2. breathe slowly and deeply to allow complete filling and emptying of the lungs
3. concentrate on having a rhythm, a pattern of breathing

Poor abdominal muscle tone can affect the efficiency of the diaphragm, an important accessory organ of respiration. An exercise that strengthens the diaphragm follows:

1. patient is seated in chair, his feet on the floor
2. patient's right hand is placed on his stomach, his left hand on his chest
3. while inhaling slowly through nose, he distends his abdomen as much as possible
4. he then exhales through pursed lips, with both hands pressing in and up on abdomen while trying to keep abdomen contracted
5. repeat as often as ordered if tolerated comfortably

It's worth emphasizing that effective coughing clears air passages of secretions. Since many elderly people have arteriosclerosis and decreased cardiac reserve, these conditions, plus increased rigidity of the rib cage, can make most coughing ineffectual. The patient simply becomes exhausted and his cough isn't beneficial. This is why simple instructions and an actual lesson in coughing are so important. The patient must make a conscious effort to activate this "cleansing" mechanism of the body.

Inhalations

The discomfort of chronic cough can often be eased by the use of steam inhalations. Electrically operated steam inhalators are used in many health care facilities and in many homes as well. Sometimes the physician will order a drug to be added to the inhalator; a common one is compound tincture of benzoin. Careful reading of instructions is important as there are many different models of inhalators on the market.

Purposes
to relieve cough and bronchial spasms
to loosen secretions
to soothe irritated and inflamed mucous membranes of the respiratory tract

Equipment
electric steam inhalator   medication as ordered

Sequence
1. identify patient; explain procedure
2. add medication (as ordered) to medicine cup of machine
3. fill water container as per manufacturer's instructions
4. keep windows and doors closed during treatment
5. time treatment; observe and record effect on patient
6. empty and clean equipment after it has cooled
7. be sure patient is dry, warm, and out of drafts
8. give oral care as necessary

   NOTES: Electric inhalators are a potential source of danger because they get very hot. The patient as well as health care personnel should be alerted to this possibility. The usual precautions in using such appliances prevail, e.g., checking for frayed cords, defective wiring, broken plugs, and so on.

   Elderly patients should be encouraged to dispose of sputum and used tissues in suitable containers. Carelessness in this respect is usually due to weakness, poor eyesight, or fatigue. When offering oral care after these inhalations, the nurse should also give the patient an opportunity to wash his hands.

Collection of Sputum Specimens

A sputum specimen may be ordered in almost any disease in which coughing is a symptom. Examples: tuberculosis, lung cancer, pneumonia, lung abscess, bronchiectasis, asthma, chronic bronchitis. The patient may need to be informed of the difference between sputum and saliva. Sputum comes from the bronchi or lungs—it isn't secreted in the mouth as is saliva, although it may be mixed with saliva. While a sputum specimen may be collected any time, two good times are early in the morning just after the patient has awakened and after postural drainage.

   Sputum specimens are ordered for diagnostic purposes. The sputum is collected in sterile sputum cups or sterile plastic sputum traps that attach to the breathing apparatus used by respiratory therapists.

Equipment

sputum container   emesis basis   tissues

Sequence
1.   identify patient, explain procedure, screen unit
2.   be sure mouth is free of food particles
3.   have patient take several deep breaths, then cough deeply and expectorate into container
4.   label container; check to see that there is no sputum on the outside; cover container
5.   nurse and patient both wash hands
6.   dispose of tissues properly
7.   give oral care as required

NOTES: It is important that the specimen be delivered to the laboratory as soon as possible. It is also helpful for the nurse to describe the specimen as to color, amount, consistency, and odor. The amount may be scant, moderate, or large; the color may be clear, yellow, rusty, greenish, blood-tinged; the consistency may be thick or thin; and the odor may be foul or odorless.

Oxygen Therapy

Hypoxia, a deficiency of oxygen, requires oxygen therapy. This therapy is ordered by the physician and is administered by nurses just like any other medication.

Some of the symptoms of hypoxia are restlessness, anxiety, and dyspnea. The skin has a blue cast (cyanosis) and the patient usually feels weak. Since breathing difficulties are so extremely frightening, these patients need as much emotional support as physical care.

Many of the newer hospitals and nursing homes have wall outlets near the patients' beds that are connected with a central oxygen supply. Others provide oxygen in cylinders or tanks.

Oxygen—colorless, odorless, and tasteless—is something we can't live without. Yet we have to be careful when living with it. Because it supports combustion, most agencies have specific rules about oxygen that have to be observed in order to avoid fires. For example, a "NO SMOKING" sign must be prominently displayed in a patient's room and on his door. If two people share a room and only one is receiving oxygen therapy, *no one* may smoke in that room. This is true even if the oxygen is used only as needed. There are many such rules and the nurse should check the policy of the agency to be sure that all necessary precautions are taken.

Oxygen is drying to the mucous membranes and therefore it is passed through either tap or distilled water before it is administered.

There are four ways of administering oxygen: by nasal cannula, nasal catheter, a face mask, and with the patient in a "tent."

When oxygen therapy is ordered, the nurse's functions are:
to administer the oxygen as ordered
to provide proper care for the patient receiving oxygen
to provide reassurance
to use adequate safety precautions

Nasal Cannula

A nasal cannula is a plastic tube with two prongs that fit into the patient's nostrils. It is secured around the patient's head with an adjustable elastic. This is a simple and comfortable way to administer oxygen and is ideal for an ambulatory patient.

1. turn on oxygen at ordered rate
2. place prongs in nostrils
3. adjust elastic, being sure it isn't too tight or causing pressure on an ear
4. clean at least once per shift
5. clean nostrils as needed

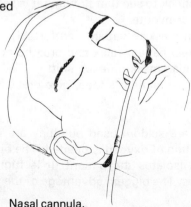

Nasal cannula.

Nasal Catheter

A catheter is used for continuous oxygen administration. It is more efficient than a cannula but not quite as comfortable. A lubricant is used on the catheter and it is passed through the nostril until it can be seen just below the uvula.

1. check that oxygen is on at rate ordered
2. remove catheter and replace it during each nursing shift, alternating nostrils if possible
3. cleanse nostril as needed with applicator moistened with water
4. observe for kinking of tubing

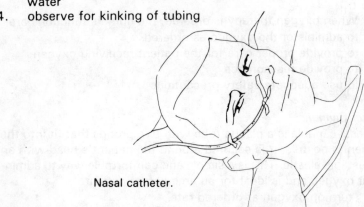

Nasal catheter.

Face Mask

A face mask is useful for administering high concentrations of oxygen. Use the following procedures:

1. check to see that flowmeter is set at ordered number of liters per minute
2. fit mask to patient comfortably
3. help patient relax and breathe normally
4. clean mask on each shift
5. wash patient's face; give oral care as necessary

Tent

Tents are seldom used but they are efficient when a high concentration of oxygen is needed. The biggest drawback to a tent is that it isolates the patient. It is frightening to patients and to families. The biggest advantage of the tent is that it allows for free movement of the patient without altering the concentration of oxygen he receives, and tents are generally used if a high concentration is going to be used for an extended period of time.

Intermittent Positive Pressure Breathing

Intermittent positive pressure breathing (IPPB) simply describes a method for forcing air and medication into the respiratory tract. It is commonly administered by a respiratory therapist for patients who need aerosol therapy or patients who need help in expectorating their secretions. Many people with COPD have trouble raising mucus from the respiratory tract and they benefit by the use of the antibiotics, expectorants, or bronchodilators used with IPPB. Respiratory therapy may combine IPPB with postural drainage, percussion, and vibration in order to relieve the breathing difficulties of these patients.

Oral Suctioning

Suctioning is done to aspirate secretions from the nose and throat and to aid in maintaining a patent airway. People who need suctioning are those who have respiratory diseases, those who are unconscious, and many aged who are too weak to bring up their own secretions.

Whenever a nurse is assigned a patient who may need suctioning, the first thing to do is to check the equipment. Is there a suction kit? Does the negative pressure gauge work? (Do you know how to turn it on?) A patient who needs suctioning usually needs it right away and the nurse must be prepared.

Equipment

suction tip, cup, glove (sterile kit)   sterile distilled water

Sequence
1. identify patient; introduce self; explain procedure
2. screen patient
3. place patient in high Fowler's position unless contraindicated
4. turn on positive pressure gauge after checking to see that there is enough distilled water in vacuum bottle under gauge

5. pour sterile water into cup from sterile kit
6. glove hand that will be touching suction tip
7. attach tubing to suction tip
8. using suction, dip tip in water to lubricate it and to see if it works (to create suction, cover opening of aspirating catheter with finger)
9. with suction *off*, gently slide aspirating catheter along side of tongue and down pharynx
10. with suction *on,* rotate catheter; suction only as long as is necessary to remove secretions
11. remove catheter while continuing suction intermittently
12. clear catheter with sterile water and repeat
13. suction as few times as possible — just enough to maintain airway

NOTES: Suctioning is irritating to pharyngeal mucosa. It stimulates secretions. It should be used sparingly. Oral care should be administered after suctioning is done.

There are several different kinds of oral suctioning apparatus. While it is a clean technique, many hospitals and nursing homes use a sterile kit and discard it after each episode of suctioning. The principles do not change, but the nurse should investigate the procedure in the hospital in which she works.

Tracheostomy Suctioning

A tracheostomy is an incision into the trachea by a surgeon in order to create an airway. It is done for several reasons: to remove an obstruction caused by a foreign body, malignancy, trauma, or respiratory disease such as croup. A tracheostomy can be permanent or temporary. The patient who has had one is very apprehensive and needs a great deal of reassurance and emotional support.

A tracheostomy set has three parts: the outer cannula; the inner cannula: the obturator.

The obturator is a guide which is placed in the outer cannula and smoothly facilitates the introduction of the outer cannula into the incision. When the surgeon is satisfied that the outer cannula is in place, the obturator is replaced by the *inner* cannula.

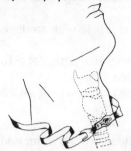

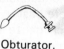
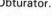
Obturator.

Inner cannula.

Outer cannula of tracheostomy
tube with tape tie.

Tracheostomy twill tape is threaded through the two slots in the
outer cannula and secured around the patient's neck. During
routine, periodic tracheostomy suctioning, the inner cannula remains in place. The technique used is described in the section on
oral suctioning. When the inner cannula is to be cleaned (as per
physician's order and PRN), then the equipment and sequence are
as follows:

Equipment

sterile suction kit   hydrogen peroxide
tracheostomy gauze   sterile water
tracheostomy twill tape   special tracheostomy brush
suture set   sterile gloves
two sterile basins   sterile applicators

Sequence
1. identify patient; introduce self; explain procedure; screen patient
2. unlock and remove soiled inner cannula; place in basin of
   hydrogen peroxide
3. clean patient's neck and remove soiled dressing as
   necessary
4. put on sterile gloves; clean incision with sterile applicators
   and sterile water
5. use suture scissors to prepare trach gauze; place gauze at
   wound site

6. scrub inner cannula with trach brush; rinse with sterile water in separate basin
7. pass trach gauze through inner cannula with Kelly forcep from suture set to dry inner cannula
8. before the inner cannula is replaced, the patient should be aspirated
9. replace and lock inner cannula
10. replace twill tapes as necessary; clean around outer cannula
11. chart time of procedure, nature of secretions, patient's tolerance of procedure

In Addition . . .

keep spare tracheostomy set at bedside for emergency
keep signal cord, writing materials at bedside
use heated mist or heated aerosol for patient
make sure patient is adequately hydrated
use only lint-free gauze for tracheostomy cleaning
chart respirations

NOTES: Although the mouth isn't sterile, the suctioning procedure is being done under surgical aseptic technique more and more frequently. The trachea is mainly free of bacteria and is *always* suctioned under the precaution of sterile technique. Another significant difference is the fact that the suction catheter is introduced only the distance of the *tracheostomy* tube, unless specifically ordered otherwise. A maximum of 15 seconds of suctioning is a good rule for both oral and tracheostomy suctioning.

REVIEW

A. Multiple Choice (Select the Best Answer)

1. Some of the energy we get from food is:
   a. changed into carbon dioxide
   b. used directly by muscle cells
   c. trapped in the alveolar sacs
   d. seldom used by the organs of respiration
2. After inhalation, carbon dioxide leaves the blood and gets collected in alveolar sacs until exhalation. This is:

    a. external respiration
    b. internal respiration
    c. extrinsic respiration
    d. intrinsic respiration

3. The partition between the thoracic cavity and the abdominal cavity is:
    a. the pleura
    b. the bronchioles
    c. the costal cartilages
    d. the diaphragm

4. The intercostals:
    a. decrease the size of the thorax upon inspiration
    b. increase the size of the thorax upon inspiration
    c. do not affect the size of the thorax
    d. are tubular structures leading to the bronchioles

5. Emphysema is characterized by:
    a. tumor growth
    b. pus in the pleural cavity
    c. overdistended alveolar sacs
    d. weight gain

B. Matching Test (Match Column 1 with Column 2)

Column 1	Column 2
a. chronic bronchitis	____6. obtained any time
b. asthma	____7. lower incidence in elderly
c. postural drainage	____8. ''cigarette'' cough
d. lung cancer	____9. before meals, at bedtime
e. sputum	___10. affected by stress, allergens

C. Briefly Answer the Following Questions

1. Describe four ways of administering oxygen
2. What does IPPB mean?
3. What is the first thing the nurse should do if assigned to a patient needing suctioning?
4. What are two disadvantages to suctioning?
5. What type of technique is used when suctioning?

10

The Digestive System

Objectives

After completing this chapter the student should be able to:

- understand the changes that occur in the digestive system with aging
- carry out a bowel retraining program
- do the procedures for enemas, tube feedings, colostomy irrigation, and oral care
- understand the measures used for inserting suppositories, for hyperalimentation, and for fecal impactions
- use the following words correctly

Vocabulary

The following words relate to the material in this chapter. Look up the ones you do not know or are not sure of.

atrophy	lateral	regressive
edentulous	metastasis	residue

exacerbate	meticulous	rugae
hypertonic	mucosa	sordes
impaction	peristalsis	stoma
intramuscular	proctoscopy	strictures

Anatomy Review

The digestive system is made up of a group of organs that take our food and then, through a series of interesting processes, get it ready for absorption into the bloodstream. Anything that isn't absorbed is excreted.

Structures and Functions

Stomach.   The stomach is a small, readily expandable sac at the end of the esophagus. Food is taken in through the mouth, chewed, swallowed, and propelled by peristaltic waves down the esophagus until it reaches the stomach. There it's stored until gastric juices and enzymes break it down further before it is passed into the small intestine. A distinctive feature of the stomach is the fact that it's lined with furrows. When we fill our stomachs, these furrows (rugae) widen and gradually disappear because the stomach has expanded. An infant's stomach has a capacity of about 60 cc, but an adult's capacity is about a liter and a half. Lining the stomach is mucous membrane, home to thousands of tiny glands that constantly secrete the gastric juice and hydrochloric acid necessary for digestion.

The Small Intestine.   This intestine is called "small" because it is slightly smaller in diameter than the large intestine. (Ordinarily you wouldn't call anything small that is 20 feet long!) The small intestine extends from the stomach and is divided into three sections: duodenum, jejunum and ileum. Intestinal digestive juices are secreted here and they also act on food to aid absorption into the blood.

Whatever is indigestible (residue) is passed through the large intestine and excreted. The sections of the seven-foot-long large intestine are: cecum (blind pouch), ascending colon, transverse colon, descending colon, sigmoid (S shaped) and rectum. Solid

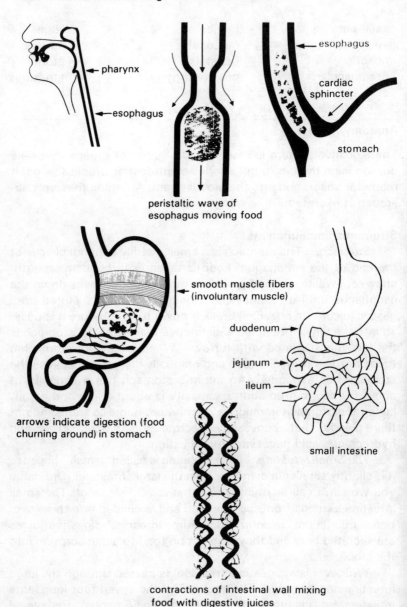

Schematic sketches of the digestive system. Courtesy Boehringer Engelheim Ltd.

wastes are called feces, and feces leave the body by way of the rectum—the last few inches of the large intestine. The external opening of the rectum is the anus. Normally, defecation, getting rid of feces, is a voluntary action.

Other structures play an important part in the digestive process, although they aren't exactly part of the digestive tract. These accessory structures are:

Teeth. The teeth prepare food for digestion by breaking it into small particles; chewing action also stimulates the flow of saliva, which in turn moistens the food and allows it to be acted on by the enzyme ptyalin, the first of many digestive enzymes it will meet on its way through the digestive tract.

Tongue. The tongue mixes food with saliva; pushes food back into the throat; and houses the invisible taste buds that are located in the tiny projections (papillae) that cover the tongue.

Salivary Glands. There are three pairs of salivary glands: the parotid (in front of ear), submandibular (under jaw), and sublingual (under tongue). They secrete saliva which contains the enzyme ptyalin.

Age-Related Changes

When learning about some of the changes in the digestive system of the elderly, it is best to begin at the beginning. One of the most obvious signs of aging besides wrinkled skin is loss of teeth.

1. *Loss of Teeth.* By middle age, 25 million people in the United States have lost half their natural teeth. Two-thirds of those over 65 have lost most of their teeth. Common dental problems of the elderly are lack of dentures, dentures that need to be fixed, and dentures that don't feel comfortable. Why don't these people take care of their teeth? Some of them *accept* the loss of teeth as a natural occurrence. Dental care is expensive and many elderly living on fixed incomes simply cannot afford, or are reluctant, to spend money for something they consider nonessential. However, the loss of teeth, and dentures that don't fit properly, make chewing food, the first step in digestion, difficult.

2. *Oral Lesions.* These go undetected because people do not see a dentist at regular intervals. Common among these le-

sions are the irritations from broken or jagged teeth and poorly fitted dentures. The steady contact of the warm pipe stem of the constant pipe smoker can produce a sore on the lip, and many of these sores become malignant.

3. *Leukoplakia.*   This common condition of the oral cavity occurs very frequently in older persons. It appears as elevated white patches on the oral mucosa and is considered a precancerous lesion. These patches may be painful but most oral lesions are not. Just because a person doesn't get a warning (pain) doesn't mean that he can afford to delay or ignore *any* oral lesion. They all must be seen and evaluated by a physician.

4. *Hypochlorhydria.*   As we age, the activity of the digestive glands in the gastric mucosa decreases. The important substance that there is less of at this time is hydrochloric acid, a secretion which prepares protein for absorption, retards the growth of bacteria, and encourages other digestive enzymes to function. Hypochlorhydria, the name given to this lessened secretion, encourages bacterial growth in the stomach and upper intestine. This may result in the increase of flatus (gas) or diarrhea.

5. *Atrophy of the Stomach.*   The aging stomach actually shrinks a bit in size and that's why small amounts of food seem to "fill up" an elderly person. Frequent small feedings may be the best way of seeing that such a patient gets all the nutrients he needs. More hospitals and nursing homes are providing a choice on their menus not only of foods but also of the portion size, which is a sensible thing to do.

6. *Slower Peristalsis.*   Think of some elderly patients you have heard complain of "gas." You already know that a decrease in hydrochloric acid secretion may be at fault. But the blame must be shared by another digestive change we will all experience if we live long enough—the slowing down of peristalsis. Therefore, it's very important to ward off that threat to good bowel hygiene by reminding the elderly patient of the importance of adequate fluid and fiber intake and reasonable exercise.

7. *Decline in Number of Taste Buds.*   As we age, the tiny

groups of cells that respond to the food they come in contact with on the tongue diminish in number. Things truly "don't taste like they used to." The decline in the number of taste buds can contribute to a decrease in appetite.

Age-Related Disorders and Diseases

1. *Diverticulosis and Diverticulitis.* It is estimated that between 20 and 25 percent of the population over the age of 40 has diverticulosis—a condition marked by the outpouching of the wall of the intestines. Tiny areas of weakness develop in the intestinal wall and these areas protrude by the hundreds. If any bowel contents becomes trapped in these pockets, infection and inflammation result. Then the condition is called diverticu*litis*. Diverticulosis may be present without symptoms and in fact it was once considered harmless. However, the possibility for obstruction is always there and diverticulitis is painful and potentially serious.

   Diverticul*osis* is treated by some physicians with a high residue, low roughage diet. Vegetables and fruits that can cause gas are omitted, as are nuts and bran. Patients may be on antispasmodics and other medications to reduce the growth of bacteria in the bowel. The overall plan is to produce a fecal mass that's soft and won't irritate the inflamed part of the bowel. The newer thinking is to place the patient on a low residue diet, monitor progress, and then advance the patient to a regular diet as tolerated. A description and sample of a low-residue diet is given in Chapter 7, page 113.

   Diverticul*itis* requires a bland, low-residue diet. If there is pain, bed rest will be ordered along with antispasmodics, tranquilizers, and stool softeners. The patient will be closely observed for exacerbation of symptoms (abdominal distention or pain; fever; nausea), as perforation of the bowel is always a possibility with diverticulitis.

2. *Hemorrhoids.* Dilated blood vessels in the anus, called hemorrhoids, may be internal or external. Nearly everyone

experiences them at one time or another. Constipation can make them very uncomfortable, but relief may be obtained by using stool softeners, witch hazel compresses, and sitz baths.

3. *Cancer.* Cancer of the colon and rectum is the most common type of cancer and it occurs frequently among the elderly population. Unfortunately, malignancies of the large bowel often go undiagnosed. Change in bowel habits, cramps, and abdominal distention all too often are accepted as the consequences of old age. Even bleeding, a startling signal to most people, is shrugged off as being caused by "piles," the lay term for hemorrhoids. The longer these symptoms are treated by home remedies, the less the chance that medical diagnosis and treatment, when they are finally given, will lead to recovery. The American Cancer Society recommends an annual proctoscopy for those over age 40. Preferred by many physicians because of its simplicity is the hematest for occult blood where a small particle of stool is placed on a disposable slide, a drop of reagent is added, and the specimen is read as being positive or negative according to a color chart.

 Over 70 percent of patients with cancer of the colon and rectum can be cured if it is diagnosed before metastasis occurs. But these people must be seen by a physician for a diagnosis to be made.

4. *Constipation.* Because constipation is such a common condition, we will deal with it at length in the following section.

Constipation*

Constipation is one of the oldest and most common medical problems and man has constantly sought means of correcting it. Legend suggests that the enema, for example, was in use long before recorded time by the ancient Chinese, Babylonians, and Egyptians. There are references to laxative compounds in the Bible,

* *This section and the following section on bowel retraining are from* Bowel Evacuation Manual and Bowel Retraining Record, *and are printed courtesy of Boeringer Ingelheim Ltd.*

and even Shakespeare mentioned purgatives in *Macbeth.*

Oddly enough, many of the drugs and formulas used by ancient civilizations for laxatives are not very different from those we use today.

In simple terms, constipation means infrequent or difficult evacuation of feces. Remember, however, that "infrequent" is relative to the individual patient. While a daily bowel movement is normal for most people, two or three times a week or even weekly may be normal for others.

It's possible for some persons who have a regular daily movement to rarely or never have a complete evacuation. Therefore, the frequency of bowel action alone is not an adequate criterion of constipation.

Constipation exists when:

1. The period between bowel actions is too long—when the interval between movements is greater than that which is normal for that individual.
2. The fecal volume is too small—when any significant amount of feces remains in the rectum after defecation, even though bowel action may be frequent.
3. The fecal consistency is too hard—so hard that the patient experiences difficulty and pain in passing the feces.

Before undertaking a program for bowel retraining, the nurse should review the common causes of constipation, which are: 1) faulty personal habits; 2) emotional factors; 3) local and systemic diseases; 4) muscular factors; 5) diet; and 6) miscellaneous other causes.

1. *Faulty Personal Habits.* If the patient consistently refuses to heed the natural urge to defecate, his awareness of rectal fullness becomes dulled and ultimately all natural periodic urge disappears more or less completely. This neglect may be the result of:
      carelessness
      demands of occupation
      stress and rush of modern living
      travel which requires abrupt adjustments to changes in time and food

(with children) the reluctance to interrupt play

neurotic habit of delay (sometimes due to faulty child-hood training)

Laxative dependence and the chronic use of harsh laxatives also contribute to the problem. After the bowel has been emptied by a purgative, it generally takes two days for fecal material to accumulate in sufficient quantity to stimulate the desire for bowel action. If the purgative is repeated in the interim, and especially if the cycle is constantly repeated, this may lead to complete loss of natural, normal bowel habits.

2. *Emotional Factors.* Hypertonic colon, a condition which produces spastic constipation, is frequently associated with emotional disturbances, especially anxiety and tension. In some people the condition is so severe that the whole colon remains in a constant state of spasm. Occasionally, this is caused by inflammatory disease.

Neurotic persons, or those obsessed with "regularity," may upset evacuation by unnecessarily taking laxatives, cathartics, or enemas. This can lead to "the laxative habit."

3. *Local and Systemic Disease.* Painful lesions such as hemorrhoids, anal fissures, anorectal lesions, and local organic lesions either within or outside the colon or rectum can make defecation painful and this contributes to constipation.

Acute illness such as cancer of the large bowel, chronic dehydration, narcotic addiction, and lead poisoning may cause constipation.

Mechanical obstructions such as tumors often cause constipation. Certain drugs, i.e., narcotic analgesics, tranquilizers and bismuth compounds also cause constipation.

4. *Muscular Factors.* Weak or displaced abdominal wall muscles may lessen the ability to increase the pressure in the abdomen sufficiently to force out the feces. Defecation becomes more difficult.

The patient with chronic pulmonary emphysema can't hold his breath long enough to cause the abdominal compression necessary for defecation.

The geriatric nurse often sees *atonic colon*—the condition of thin, weak colonic musculature and ineffective peristaltic contractions. It's quite common in the elderly and in those with chronic debilitating diseases.

5. *Diet.* Food intake lacking in bulk or fluids can cause constipation. When food bulk is too small to cause normal distention, peristaltic movements become sluggish. Inadequate fluids cause the food residue to become hard and this is more difficult to move along the alimentary canal.

    Persons on rigid reducing diets often suffer from constipation because there is a lack of bulk.

    A patient who is NPO, as, for example, after surgery, usually will not have regular bowel movements until normal function of body organs occurs.

    Some people (especially infants) become constipated from milk, since the large amount of casein in cow's milk tends to produce hard, firm stools. Milk products, i.e., cheeses, ice cream and so on, can also be constipating in certain individuals.

6. *Miscellaneous.* During pregnancy, as the uterus enlarges, and later, as the fetal head presses down on the rectum, the bowel is compressed and the space for the passage of bowel contents is limited.

    Patients confined to bed for prolonged periods of time are inactive. Forced immobilization leads to muscle weakness and sluggish bowels, making complete evacuation difficult.

    Certain intestinal disorders (megacolon and congenital abnormalities) may also cause constipation.

For nutritional suggestions for overcoming constipation, see Chapter 7, pages 107 to 109.

When food and good hygiene aren't enough to establish and maintain good bowel habits, the physician may order thorough bowel cleansing, i.e., laxatives, cathartics, and enemas. These bowel evacuants work in different ways and have advantages and disadvantages. Enemas are discussed on pages 179-184.

About Laxatives

1. *Bulk Laxatives.*   The bulk laxatives may be divided into two groups: the saline laxatives and the hydrophilic colloids. All the bulk laxatives increase the bulk of the stool by increasing its water content. They reach this goal by different means, however.

    The *saline laxatives* form a concentrated saline solution of high osmotic pressure in the intestine and actually draw fluid from the intestinal wall by osmosis. Examples:

magnesium hydroxide (milk of magnesia)	magnesium carbonate
	magnesium oxide
magnesium sulfate (Epsom salt)	sodium sulfate
	sodium phosphate
magnesium citrate	

    CAUTION: Saline laxatives may be violent in action: watery stools, colicky pain, and dehydration often follow their use.

    The *hydrophilic colloids* simply absorb water from the intestinal contents. Generally, they are able to absorb amounts of liquid up to about ten times their own weight. They are more gentle in action but are seldom effective in relieving acute, severe constipation. Examples: agar, psyllium, manna, bran, and methylcellulose.

    CAUTION: These laxatives require that the patient drink sufficient water to insure effectiveness of the product.

2. *Detergent Stool Softeners.*   Detergent stool softeners are essentially wetting agents. They promote both the retention of water and the emulsification of fats and are quite effective in insuring a soft stool. Although they provide a soft stool, it's often necessary to take them for two or three days before having a satisfactory bowel movement. Some examples are: dioctyl, sodium succinate, and propylene oxide.

3. *Emollient Laxatives.*   These laxatives are simple lubricants—mineral oil and some vegetable oils. They have a mild effect, that is, they do not produce cramping. They are extremely useful in keeping the stool soft when straining could be hazardous, i.e., in aneurysm, cerebral hemorrhage, and after hemorrhoidectomy.

A problem with the emollients is that there is sometimes embarrassing leakage through the anal sphincter. Also, habitual use of mineral oil may interfere with the absorption of the fat soluble vitamins A, D, and K.

4. *Contact Laxative.*Bisacodyl (Dulcolax) is known as a contact laxative because of its particular mode of action. It takes effect when it comes in contact with the colonic mucosa where it stimulates nerve endings in the intestinal wall. The nerve impulses produced reflexly stimulate peristaltic movement in the colon. This peristalsis propels the mass of wastes through the large intestine to the colon and rectum where it brings about a natural urge to defecate.

As with any laxative, there may be some abdominal cramping.

About Laxative and Evacuant Suppositories
Like the oral tablets, Dulcolax suppositories act when they come in contact with the colonic mucosa of the intestinal wall and produce evacuation in the same way. They are faster acting than the tablets, however, usually producing an effect within 15 minutes to one hour. Many nursing homes and hospitals use these suppositories before or in place of using enemas.

Glycerin irritates the rectum mechanically. The bowel attempts to eliminate the irritation by diluting it with a secretion of fluid. The fluid acts as a lubricant and liquefacient and a fecal discharge follows. Glycerin suppositories used occasionally aren't harmful but if they're depended on habitually, they may injure the mucous membrane.

Carbon dioxide suppositories release the gas in the lower part of the colon to create pressure and stimulate the peristaltic and defecation reflexes. Usually the effect is in the lower rectum only.

Nursing Measures and Procedures

Bowel Retraining
Bowel retraining is needed in many cases of chronic constipation. These patients may include geriatric cases, patients with colos-

tomies, and stroke patients with atonic or spastic conditions. A routine bowel retraining program can generally be used in such cases, keeping in mind that in spastic constipation the physician will often prescribe or make some changes in the retraining program.

Beginning the Program

1. obtain the physician's order
2. gain the patient's cooperation and understanding; explain the program and encourage full participation
3. obtain a bowel history of the patient's food habits, fluid intake, and use of laxatives
4. perform a manual examination of the rectum if necessary (if an impaction is present, follow agency policy for removal)
5. evaluate other associated factors; example, decubitus ulcers, senility, patient's motivation and acceptance
6. start the training with a clean bowel

Guidelines for the Program

1. establish a regular evacuation time (daily or on alternate days)
2. provide for maximum mobility of the patient; encourage exercise within limits permitted by the physician and tolerated by the patient
3. maintain complete records; record all results observed on each shift for each patient in the program
4. see that the patient takes adequate fluids
5. provide accessory physical facilities (privacy, commodes, toilet extenders, footstools, or anything else to make the patient comfortable)
6. persevere — anticipate lapses during the first 10 days
7. review the progress of the program with the physician, the staff, and the patient

Daily Procedure

1. the diet should be prescribed by the physician and should be

		eating habits (heavy, medium, light)	physical exercise (good, poor, none)	equipment required or facility used (diaper, bedpan, toilet)	time & number of Dulcolax* suppositories	confirmed time of evacuation	stool condition (hard, soft, fluid) and quantity	remarks
date	approx. fluid intake							

BOWEL RETRAINING RECORD   **Sample of completed chart**

patient's name: John Doe   ward: F-3   date program started: 6/5

patient's previous bowel pattern: frequency: Daily   time: A.M.

present bowel pattern: ☐ constipation   ☒ incontinence

    ☐ high impaction   ☐ low impaction

problem arising from: ☐ age   ☐ drugs   ☐ neurological

    ☐ psychiatric   ☒ CVA   other (specify)

time of scheduled defecation: ☒ after breakfast   ☐ after lunch   ☐ after dinner

date	approx. fluid intake	eating habits	physical exercise	equipment/facility used	time & number of suppositories	confirmed time of evacuation	stool condition	remarks
6/5	400cc 650cc	medium		bedpan	1 supp. 9 A.M.	9:16 A.M.	fluid	slight cramping
	300cc 800cc	medium				7:45 P.M.	fluid	unscheduled defecation
	750cc	medium	none					
6/6	500cc	medium		bedpan	1 supp. 9 A.M.	9:22 A.M.	semi-fluid	
	1200cc	heavy						
	1100cc	heavy	poor					

A bowel retraining record. Courtesy Boeringer Ingelheim Ltd.

well-balanced, with no food between meals; all meals should be served at a regular time each day

2. fluid intake per day should be 2,500 to 3,000 cc; prune juice, two to four ounces, is started on the first day without a stool or if the stool is exceptionally firm; output should be fairly comparable to intake

3. use of bowel evacuant:

   a) daily (after breakfast), depending on the pattern of the individual patient; insert Dulcolax suppository as high as finger will reach into the rectum past the internal sphincter

   b) timing: note how much time elapses until the patient has a desire to evacuate; it will vary with each patient—usually from 15 minutes to an hour; *keep records*

   c) place patient on commode or assist him to bathroom;

with nonambulatory patient, use bedpan or diaper if necessary

d)   the presence of liquid stool or "oozing" is often a sign of impaction; check the patient digitally and follow the agency's procedures

e)   if liquid stools continue and no impaction is found, give four ounces tap water enema for three or four days until normal stools are obtained; report progress to physician

Termination of Program

1.   continue daily training procedures for 14 to 21 days
2.   gradually discontinue Dulcolax tablets or suppositories; goal of program is regular bowel habits for the patient without laxative support

Fecal Incontinence

While fecal incontinence is not a true form of constipation, it should be mentioned here in relation to bowel retraining. In plegic patients, patients with spinal cord injury or CVA, bowel retraining is an important consideration in rehabilitation.

Where bowel retraining is impossible, regulation of bowel habit is usually possible. Many hospitals and nursing homes have

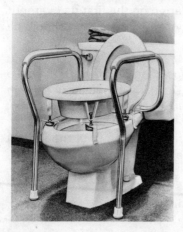

Raised toilet seat with slip-on brackets and toilet safety frame. Ideal for arthritic, stroke, or fractured-hip patients and also for weak patients. Courtesy of Lumex, Inc.

found that their patients are helped by the administration of a suppository to bring about a daily bowel evacuation. In this way the patient doesn't have frequent, uncontrolled bowel movements during the day.

When the bisacodyl suppository is given after breakfast, it usually produces a response in 15 minutes to an hour. Bowel management can be completed in the morning.

Fecal Impactions

It is possible for a large, dry mass of feces to obstruct the rectum. This impaction will irritate the rectal mucosa and the patient will have oozing of liquid stool or diarrhea, but the impaction will remain unless manually removed. The nurse may try an oil retention enema to soften the fecal mass. If this is not effective, it may be necessary to insert a well-lubricated, gloved finger into the rectum *very gently* to break up the fecal impaction. This procedure is extremely uncomfortable and the patient must be watched closely for untoward effects such as pallor, diaphoresis, rapid pulse, rectal bleeding, and so on. If any of these symptoms occur, stop the procedure.

NOTE: Enemas and manual removal of fecal impactions are done only on a physician's order, and in some health care facilities they are done by physicians or RNs only. Be sure to know the written policy where you practice nursing.

Giving Enemas

The oldest means of cleansing the bowel requires the introduction of fluid into the rectum. The efficacy of the enema depends on the substance used.

1. saline enema—draws water into the colon, increasing pressure on its walls and inducing a reaction in the form of defecation.
2. oil enema—lubricates the rectum and softens feces, thus facilitating defecation.
3. soapsuds enema—irritates the colon, causing it to react and produce defecation.

NOTES: Even though enemas have been popular for centuries, their use shouldn't be taken lightly. It's a serious procedure. Even a tap water enema may be dangerous, especially in infants and young children. If the enema is too hot, the intestinal wall can be injured. Too much salt may cause inflammation of the colon, and even a soapsuds enema may cause some inflammation. *Laxatives and enemas should never be given when there is nausea, vomiting, or abdominal pain.*

Basically, there are two categories of enemas; retention and nonretention. The common retention enemas are the oil retention enema and the Harris drip. The nonretention enemas are the cleansing enemas, i.e., the tap water enema, the soapsuds enema, and the commercially prepared hypertonic solution in a plastic disposable squeeze bottle.

Oil Retention Enema

Purposes
to lubricate the rectum and lower bowel
to aid in the removal of feces

Equipment
lubricant   bedpan
disposable protective pad   bath blanket
                                                 toilet tissue

Sequence
1. identify patient; introduce self; explain procedure; screen patient
2. fanfold top bedding to foot of bed, cover patient with bath blanket
3. place patient in left lateral position, knees flexed
4. tuck protective pad under hips
5. lubricate enema tip, insert into anus about four inches
6. instill oil slowly, encouraging patient to mouth breathe and ask him to retain the oil for at least 30 minutes   apply pressure over anus for a minute or two after withdrawing enema tip; replace bed covers

7.   record type of enema, amount of solution, and patient's reaction

ADDITIONAL INFORMATION: The oil retention enema is usually ordered if a patient is severely constipated, has painful hemorrhoids, or has had a fecal impaction removed. In all cases, the nurse should be as gentle as possible in carrying out the procedure. Frequently the oil enema is followed, after a given period of time, by a cleansing enema. This is also ordered by the physician. The nurse then assists the patient to the bathroom if permitted, or positions him on a bedpan with the curtains drawn and with toilet tissue and a call light at hand. Aftercare is administered as necessary.

When bowel evacuation occurs, the nurse charts the time of the procedure and the amount and type of enema solution. Results of enemas should be documented: amount, color, consistency, and patient's reaction.

NOTE: There are some commonsense adjustments that will have to be made if the person giving the enema is inexperienced with elderly people. For example, the preferred left-side lying position may be uncomfortable for someone with arthritis, contractures, and so on. The patient may have to be placed on his back and supported with pillows. If the patient is incontinent, gloves must be worn and the enema must be administered on the bedpan. Even if the patient is confined to bed, better results are achieved if an effort is made to get him up on a commode.

Harris Drip Enema

The Harris drip is a retention enema that is given to help the patient expel flatus (gas) and relieve abdominal distention. Properly done, it provides tremendous relief from the intense discomfort of gas pains that even analgesics seldom relieve. (Analgesics relieve the pain, but that bloated, uncomfortable feeling remains.)

What happens when the drip is given is this: as the enema bag is raised, a small quantity of water is allowed to flow into the rectum. Then, as the bag is lowered below the level of the bed, the solution, plus the gas in the form of bubbles, flows back out of the patient into the enema bag. This is repeated for about 15 minutes until gradually the patient's gas pain is relieved. The nurse will adapt the length of the procedure to the patient's tolerance.

Purposes
to expel flatus
to relieve abdominal distention

Equipment

plastic enema bag	disposable protective pad
lubricant	bath blanket
500 cc tap water (or the pres-	bedpan
cribed amount of solution)	toilet tissue
105-110°F	

Sequence
  1. identify patient; introduce self; explain procedure; screen patient
  2. fanfold top bedding to bottom of bed, cover patient with the bath blanket
  3. place patient in left lateral position, knees flexed
  4. tuck protective pad under hips
  5. lubricate enema tip and insert tubing four inches into anus
  6. lower enema bag below level of bed (the inserted tube may irritate the lower bowel enough to encourage passage of flatus)
  7. raise bag about 18 inches above the anus and allow 50-100 cc of solution to flow into patient
  8. repeat raising and lowering of enema bag until nearly all solution has been administered or until patient experiences relief from distention; pinch off tubing before withdrawing
  9. provide aftercare of patient as needed
 10. record time of procedure, type and amount of solution, reaction of patient

ADDITIONAL INFORMATION: In the past there have been other kinds of retention enemas, for example, nutritive enemas, medication enemas, and anthelmintic (pertaining to parasites) enemas. Over the years, however, more efficient means have been developed for the problems these enemas used to treat. Intramuscular injections and intravenous medications are commonplace in all health care facilities. But it wasn't always so. At one time a frequent route of administration was the rectal instillation. If the patient couldn't take an oral medication, the physician might order it rectally. It helps the nurse develop a sense of history to learn a bit about the evolution of some procedures.

Nonretention or Cleansing Enema

A cleansing enema is given to rid the colon and lower bowel of feces. A physician's order is necessary for the tap water, soapsuds, or commercially packaged hypertonic solution. (This last increases the amount of fluid in the colon as it draws fluid from the body, which in turn stimulates peristalsis.)

It's unfortunate that most procedures are done at the convenience of the staff, not the patient. However, an enema should never be administered too close to mealtimes, visiting hours, or bedtime.

Purposes
to empty the rectum of feces
to relieve distention

Equipment
either tap water or soapsuds, as per physician's order, 105-110°F, plastic enema bag (or irrigating can with tubing and clamp)
lubricant
bed pan, toilet tissue
bath blanket
disposable protective pad

Sequence
1. identify patient; introduce self; explain procedure; screen patient
2. fanfold top bedding to foot of bed; cover patient with bath blanket
3. place patient in left lateral position, knees flexed
4. tuck protective pad under hips
5. lubricate enema tip, insert into anus about four inches
6. slowly introduce solution into rectum with the enema bag at a height of about 18 inches above the anus
7. instruct patient to take deep breaths during procedure and reassure him that if cramping is a problem you will stop the procedure until cramping subsides
8. when most of solution has been given, clamp off tubing and withdraw it
9. position patient on bedpan, leave toilet tissue and call light within reach, OR
10. assist patient to bathroom and instruct him not to flush the toilet until contents have been observed
11. aftercare of patient as needed; use of room deodorizer as needed
12. record: time of procedure; amount and type of solution used; reaction of patient; amount, color, and consistency of results of enema

MORE ABOUT ENEMAS: Beginning students often ask, "Can I perforate the rectal mucosa by giving an enema from too high a level or by giving it too fast?" The answer is a qualified no. To be sure, the rectal mucosa of an elderly patient is probably thinner than that of a younger adult, but perforation won't take place unless there is a stricture or other type of anomaly in the rectum. Perforation might also take place if a hard or sharp instrument was carelessly used, but not from the flow of water alone. However, if an enema is given too fast or too high, the patient will complain of abdominal cramping and most likely will not be able to hold the enema. The nurse will find herself with a bed to change.

Rectal Tube

Occasionally abdominal distention due to flatus may be relieved by using a rectal tube. The tube irritates the lower bowel just enough to stimulate peristalsis and cause the flatus to be expelled. Usually this procedure does not require a written order by the physician but hospital policy should be verified.

Purposes

to expel flatus
to relieve abdominal distention

Equipment

rectal tube OR plastic enema bag
ABD pad or 5 x 9 combine; rubber band
lubricant
disposable protective pad

Sequence

1. identify patient; introduce self; explain procedure; screen patient
2. position patient on left side, knees flexed
3. secure dressing to rectal tube with rubber band, lubricate tip, OR lubricate tip of plastic enema bag tubing
4. uncover patient just enough to expose anus
5. insert tube four inches into anus while instructing patient to lie quietly and take deep breaths
6. keep tube in place 20 minutes
7. remove tube and clean it as per hospital policy
8. aftercare of patient as necessary
9. record time, procedure, patient's reaction to procedure, and what was observed, i.e., relief of flatus, feces expelled, fecal fluid expelled, and so on

Occasionally a student will ask if it ever happens that "what goes in (solution) doesn't come out." Yes, that does happen. And when it does, the nurse uses siphonage. The patient who doesn't expel an enema is going to be uncomfortable and anxious. If a rectal tube is inserted in the anus and a small amount of warm water is allowed to flow through the tube, the retained solution can then be drained off into a bedpan. Siphonage is created because fluids flow from an area of high pressure to an area of low pressure. Offer the patient a bedpan or assist him to a commode if it is permitted. Record the procedure as "siphonage" and observe the amount of solution returned, the color, and the consistency.

Rectal Suppositories

A suppository is a small cone-shaped semisolid containing a medication in a base (glycerin or cocoa butter) that melts at body temperature. Because suppositories melt so easily, they are usually kept in the refrigerator. There are rectal suppositories and vaginal suppositories. Rectal suppositories may be ordered to relieve pain, soothe the rectum, or to cause a bowel evacuation. The rectal suppositories that cause a bowel evacuation release a gas as they melt. This in turn stimulates peristalsis and eventually causes a bowel movement. They are an alternative to enemas.

Purposes
to cause a bowel evacuation
to relieve abdominal distention due to flatus and constipation

Equipment
disposable protective pad   suppository
finger cot or disposable rubber glove   lubricant

Sequence
1.   identify patient; introduce self; explain procedure; screen patient
2.   place patient in left lateral position, knees flexed
3.   expose patient just enough to tuck protective pad under hips and visualize anus
4.   put on finger cot (or glove); lubricate suppository and index finger
5.   insert suppository gently until pressure of the inner anal sphincter is felt upon index finger
6.   apply external pressure over anus after suppository is in

serted until the patient's urge to expel the suppository has passed
7.   record time of procedure and results obtained

NOTE: The attention of the elderly is frequently focused on their bowels—sometimes to the point of anxiety. Large doses of patience and understanding are needed. With a view toward avoiding dependency on enemas and laxatives, the nurse might create learning opportunities for patients by observing their eating habits and then by discussing the relationship of nutrition, adequate fluids, and reasonable exercise to healthful elimination patterns.

Feeding
Even people who can feed themselves may need some assistance if they are confined to bed. For example, before a tray is served, does a dressing need to be changed? Should oral care be given? Are the patient's hands washed? Is the patient in a position for a comfortable pleasant meal? Preparing a patient for mealtime includes mental as well as physical preparation. An unclut-

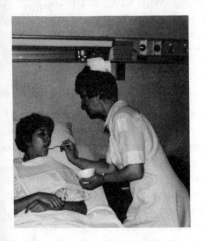 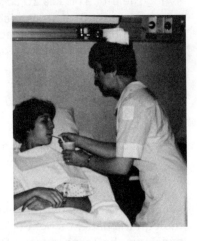

One nurse practices her feeding skills on another in a laboratory setting. The "patient" soon finds out how important good feeding skills are.

tered, tension-free environment is necessary because food is an important part of the overall care plan.

If the patient is to be fed, first check to see if he may receive a tray. Then verify that the diet to be served is the correct diet. Place the tray on an overbed table and raise the head of the bed as necessary. Protect the top bedding with a towel and place a napkin under the patient's chin. Prepare the foods by pouring hot liquids, buttering bread, and cutting meat. Permit the patient to hold the bread or to feed himself if he is able to. Offer fluids and foods in a slow, relaxed manner. Conversation should be quiet and uncontroversial.

Blind patients who can feed themselves should have their trays explained to them, using the hands of a clock as fixation points. For example, "Your juice is at 12 o'clock, tea at 12:15," and so on. Encourage the patient's enjoyment of the meal by commenting that "the roll looks crispy" or "the soup seems tasty." If there are nuts in the cupcake, it's a good idea to say so. People like to know what they are eating.

Often very elderly, regressed patients neither suck from a straw nor accept food from a spoon. The nurse will find a feeding syringe helpful. This is a 20 cc syringe with a two-inch-long rubber tube on the end of it. Pureed foods and fluids are offered by syringe, thus maintaining adequate intake.

Charting should include approximate amounts of solids and fluids the patient consumes.

Nasogastric Tube Feeding
Many patients have problems chewing or swallowing. Sometimes these problems prevent them from eating normally. For example, stroke victims, unconscious patients, people too depressed to eat, and patients who have had extensive head and neck surgery all present severe feeding problems. In these cases, a nasogastric tube feeding may be ordered. A nasogastric tube (Levin's tube) is a long plastic or rubber tube with a narrow lumen that is inserted through the patient's right or left nostril, down past the pharynx, and down the esophagus until it reaches the stomach. The patient is fed a formula or a blenderized diet through the tube, which is usually kept in place for several days at a time. Usually a nurse is

assigned to do this. If an aide, orderly, or health assistant has this assignment, detailed instructions as well as nursing supervision is necessary.

Other uses for a nasogastric tube are:

1. Stomach contents may be aspirated for a laboratory examination.
2. Surgeons may order the stomach contents to be aspirated before doing major abdominal surgery in order to keep fluids and gas from accumulating in the stomach.
3. Gastric lavage is done through a nasogastric tube when harmful substances have been ingested.

Purpose
to provide nourishment when ordinary means of feeding are
   impossible

Equipment

Asepto syringe or	napkin
50 cc syringe	glass of warmed water (105° F)
towel	prescribed feeding, warmed to 105°F

Sequence

1. identify patient; introduce self; explain procedure; screen patient
2. place patient in Fowler's position if he can tolerate this
3. protect gown and bedclothes with towel
4. remove clamp from nasogastric tube and with syringe aspirate a few cc of gastric contents to insure correct location of tube
5. using Asepto syringe or 50 cc syringe allow 30 cc water at room temperature to flow into tube *via gravity*
6. follow this with prescribed feeding, slowly. Avoid introduction of air by keeping syringe full at all times and controlling feeding by raising and lowering syringe (about 30 cc per minute is comfortable for the patient)
7. follow tube feeding with 30 cc of water at room temperature in order to clear tubing.

Gastrostomy Tube Feeding

A gastrostomy is an operation in which an artificial opening is made into the stomach to allow for the administration of fluids and foods. A rubber or plastic tube is introduced through the abdominal wall into the stomach and secured there. A gastrostomy tube feeding is done the same way as a nasogastric tube feeding. Remember to provide privacy. An important nursing measure to remember when caring for the gastrostomy patient is to keep the skin around the opening of the abdominal wall meticulously clean. (Be sure the clamp is on the tube after feeding to prevent leakage of gastric contents!) Three hundred to 500 ml is the usual amount given for each meal. A feeding takes 10 to 15 minutes. Also, the patient who has a gastrostomy probably hasn't been taking much, if anything, by mouth for quite a while and he's often dehydrated. Give frequent, thorough oral care.

Tube feedings are unnatural, distasteful ways of receiving one's nourishment, and the nurse's pleasant, matter-of-fact attitude can go a long way toward reassuring the patient.

Hyperalimentation (Total Parenteral Nutrition)

Hyperalimentation is a means of providing the body with nutrients intravenously. This means of nutritional support is used when oral feedings or tube feedings are contraindicated.

The prescribed solution contains more calories than ordinary IVs and is most frequently administered through the subclavian vein which leads to the superior vena cava.

The nurse's responsibility is to maintain sterile aseptic technique, and to be sure that the indwelling catheter is patent and that the solution is infusing at the prescribed drip rate. Accurate recording of hyperalimentation is also a nursing duty.

Colostomy Irrigation

A colostomy irrigation may be compared to an enema. The difference is that the solution is introduced through an artificial anus called a stoma that has been created on the abdominal wall. Colostomy surgery is done to relieve obstructions or to rest the bowel, and the stoma may be temporary or permanent. Of course, the initial psychological trauma is just as bad in either case when

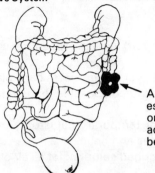

A colostomy. This surgically established fistula between the colon and the surface of the abdomen acts as an artificial anus and may be either temporary or permanent.

the patient actually sees his feces leaving his body by way of an abdominal stoma. A temporary colostomy may be "double barreled," that is, with two stomas. One of them is called the *distal* opening and the other the *proximal* opening. The physician indicates which stoma is to be irrigated. The stoma that's not irrigated drains some mucus.

Irrigations usually begin about the fourth or fifth day postoperatively. While successful irrigations depend on several things, regularity and diet should be emphasized. Irrigations are best done after a meal because eating stimulates peristalsis and bowel evacuation. Diet will affect the functioning of a colostomy and the patient will simply note the foods that cause him discomfort.

Postoperative colostomy dressings will have to be changed frequently. The attitude and attention of the nurse can affect the motivation of her patient, as the odor and the distress of wet dressings and full colostomy bags are disheartening.

Purpose
to irrigate the bowels of a patient who has a colostomy

Equipment
commercial colostomy irrigation
    set or disposable enema bag
colostomy irrigating pouch
temporary colostomy bag
disposable protective pads
lubricant
finger cot
bath blanket

solution as ordered
dressings as needed
bedpan
tincture of benzoin spray (or
other skin preparation)
paper bag for discards
two emesis basins

Sequence
1. identify patient; introduce self; explain procedure; screen patient
2. fanfold top bedding and cover patient with bath blanket
3. position patient on side with disposable pads underneath him
4. remove soiled dressings or temporary colostomy bag
5. clean skin with warm water and soap
6. fill irrigation set with prescribed solution; let all air out of tubing
7. put finger cot on; lubricate cot if stoma is to be dilated *or* just lubricate tip of tubing
8. encourage patient to hold the emesis basin close to the body just below the stoma if he is able to
9. insert tubing three to four inches into stoma and allow solution to flow in slowly. If patient complains of cramping, stop and wait until cramps subside before resuming procedure
10. remind patient confined to bed to lie quietly while returns are emptying into emesis basin.
11. if irrigation is taking place in the bathroom with patient sitting on the toilet, direct the open end of the irrigating bag into the toilet and be sure patient is warm and comfortable; observe patient for weakness, dizziness; results take about 20 minutes on the average, but 45 minutes to an hour isn't unusual
12. when irrigation is over, discard disposables into discard bag
13. wash and pat skin dry; hold gauze square over stoma and spray skin with skin preparation of choice
14. inspect adhesive surface of temporary colostomy bag to be sure it will fit snugly to the area
15. custom fit colostomy bag over stoma as indicated by directions; secure bottom of bag with rubber band
16. replace linens as needed; clean utensils
17. aftercare of patient as needed
18. record time of procedure, returns, patient's tolerance of irrigation

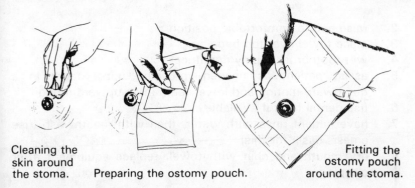

Cleaning the skin around the stoma.   Preparing the ostomy pouch.   Fitting the ostomy pouch around the stoma.

Routine Oral Care

Keeping the teeth and mouth clean slows the growth of disease-producing microorganisms, stimulates a flagging appetite, and refreshes the patient. Besides such common oral problems as infection and decay, the nurse may also observe bleeding, sordes, and irritation due to improperly fitted dentures or jagged teeth. These observations should be recorded and reported so the proper action may be taken.

Most of us take brushing our teeth for granted. But for a patient confined to the hospital, particularly a geriatric patient, this activity of daily living requires modification.

Purposes
to keep the teeth and mouth clean
to stimulate appetite
to refresh the patient

Equipment

face towel	paper cups	mouthwash
toothbrush		water
dentifrice		emesis basin

Sequence
1.   identify patient; introduce self; explain procedure; screen patient

2. raise bed to comfortable position
3. place towel over top bedding
4. wet toothbrush; apply dentifrice
5. assist patient as needed, brushing upper teeth in a downward motion and lower teeth in an upward motion
6. use dental floss if available
7. have patient rinse with water, then with mouthwash (use emesis basin for this)
8. dry mouth and chin with towel; replace equipment after cleaning

Special Oral Care

If the patient is very weak or is unconscious, special oral care is needed. The equipment may be modified to include a padded tongue blade and a lemon/glycerin swab or toothette if a brush bruises the gums. (Caution: observe patient closely to see that the toothette isn't bitten off!)

The sequence is the same as in Steps 1 through 4. Of course, the patient can't rinse his mouth, so several moistened swabs or a few padded tongue blades may have to be used to thoroughly clean and rinse the mouth. After the mouth and chin are dried, lubricant is applied.

Special mouth care should be administered several times a day to prevent sordes, the accumulation of brown crusts on the lips and teeth.

Denture Care

Dentures should be brushed the same as teeth—after early AM care, after each meal, and before bedtime. Since many people are self-conscious about dentures, privacy is important. If the patient is giving himself oral care, simply draw the curtain and see that the necessary equipment is at hand.

Equipment
denture brush
commercial denture cleanser (regular
    dentifrice may be substituted)
emesis basin

small towel
paper cups
water
mouthwash

Sequence

1. identify patient; introduce self; explain procedure; screen patient
2. place patient in comfortable position; cover top bedding with towel
3. to remove dentures for helpless patient:
    hold upper denture between thumb and forefinger
    loosen denture gently to release suction and take out of mouth
    place in denture cup or emesis basin
    repeat for lower denture
4. carry dentures to sink and brush either over a basin of water or over a towel (a safety precaution in case nurse drops dentures)
5. use denture brush designed for small crevices
6. apply denture adhesive if needed
7. return dentures to patient either by way of denture cup or by handling with a paper towel
8. dry dentures are always moistened with cold water before placing them in a patient's mouth

NOTES: Dentures are easily lost. Many times they have been placed in a pillow case or drawer or on a tray. Many nursing homes have instituted the practice of engraving names on dental plates to help identify them correctly. Dentures should always be placed in labeled denture cups when they are not being worn.

Some other aids to oral care are: baking soda (bicarbonate) as a substitute dentifrice, and sodium perborate or glyoxide for rinsing the mouth in severe cases of oral irritation.

REVIEW

A. Multiple Choice (Select the Best Answer)

1. The wavelike movements that occur in the esophagus and small and large intestines are called:
    a. rugae
    b. ptyalin
    c. flatus
    d. peristalsis

   2. An obvious sign of aging is:
      a. wrinkling of skin
      b. arteriosclerosis
      c. stomach atrophy
      d. achlorhydria
   3. A useful step toward decreasing dependence on laxatives is:
      a. increased fluid intake
      b. decreased exercise
      c. increased bedrest
      d. periodic enemas
   4. A patient who might have a swallowing problem would be:
      a. a patient on bedrest
      b. a patient in traction
      c. a stroke victim
      d. a colostomy patient
   5. Arrange the following procedure in consecutive order. When preparing a patient for a nasogastric tube feeding:
      a. allow the solution to flow in via gravity
      b. aspirate a few cc of gastric contents
      c. place patient in Fowler's position
      d. screen patient

B. Matching Test (Match Column 1 with Column 2)

Column 1	Column 2
a. rugae	_____6. small herniations of intestinal wall
b. parotid gland	_____7. elevated white patches on oral mucosa
c. leukoplakia	_____8. furrows in stomach
d. diverticulosis	_____9. used if enema isn't expelled
e. siphonage	_____10. located in front of ear

C. Briefly Answer the Following Questions

   1. What are the signs of a fecal impaction?
   2. How does a Harris drip differ from other enemas?
   3. What are some reasons for bowel problems in the aged?
   4. What is a colostomy and why is it performed?
   5. Give four steps in a bowel training program.

11

The Musculoskeletal System

Objectives
After completing this chapter the student should be able to:

- list the major changes that occur in the aging musculoskeletal system
- describe the functions of the musculoskeletal system
- carry out nursing measures and procedures for patients in traction, casts, and restraints
- understand the uses of prostheses, crutches, braces, walkers, and canes
- understand how crutch-walking gaits are taught
- position patients correctly
- use the following words correctly

Vocabulary
The following words relate to the material in this chapter. Look up the ones you do not know or are not sure of.

alignment   contracture   lactic acid

arthroplasty	facies	plantar flexion
articulate	gait	remission
chronic	hypostatic	systemic

Anatomy Review

Structures and functions

Muscles.   Muscles are generally classified as voluntary and involuntary. Voluntary muscles are also referred to as skeletal muscles since they are attached to bones. They pull on the bones and make the body move. These muscles are constructed of striated (striped) muscle fibers.

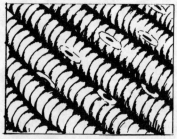

Striated muscle.

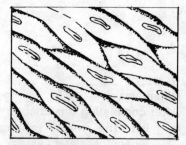

Smooth muscle.

Involuntary muscles (smooth or visceral muscles) make up walls of the intestines, blood vessels and abdominal organs. They are built of small, spindle-shaped muscle fibers and are not striated. The heart is made up of cardiac muscle which is a type of involuntary muscle.

As we use our skeletal muscles, a waste product called lactic acid builds up. This eventually tires us so that we have to sleep. After a hard day of pulling on the bones, making the body move, and keeping the body in position, our muscles become fatigued and we feel weary. Visceral muscles which work more slowly and steadily and in a more or less regular pattern with rest periods between contractions, aren't affected by fatigue. These muscles work automatically whereas the skeletal muscles will not work without express stimulation from motor nerves.

Bones. Two-thirds of the material that make up the bones consists of minerals, mainly calcium and phosphorous. The remaining third is fibrous protein. Bones are spongy on the inside and extremely hard (compact) on the outside. They provide the supporting structure for muscles, tendons, and ligaments.

Almost every bone in the body articulates with another bone; that is, each bone functions with another bone to produce movements. These articulations are called joints.

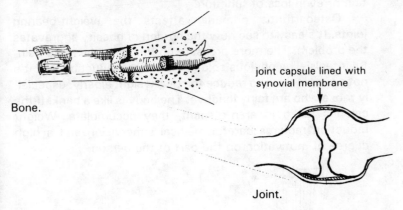

Bone.

joint capsule lined with synovial membrane

Joint.

Cartilage. The articulations at the ends of bones are covered with smooth cartilage which provides flexibility. Cartilage is also found in the rib cage, where flexibility is very important to breathing.

Joints. Some joints, such as those in the skull, don't move, but most joints are freely movable. Movable joints are contained in a joint capsule made up of fibrous connective tissue which is lined with a slippery synovial membrane. This membrane secretes synovial fluid which prevents friction during movement. The capsule covers the ends of the two articulating bones like a sheath.

Joints have two functions: to hold bones together and to provide for a range of movement between these bones. As we age, however, several problems may develop which bring discomfort and impaired function to our joints. Among them are the adhesions that form between the cartilage and overgrowth of bone at the joint edges.

Age-Related Changes in the Musculoskeletal System

1. *Joint Degeneration.* More than 90 percent of adults over the age of 65 have some degree of degenerative joint disease (osteoarthritis) as a result of the continuous wear and tear on the joints over the years. Usually, but not always, joints become painful and/or stiff. Cartilage thins, bones overgrow, spurs form, and the ultimate result can be limitation or even loss of function.

    Osteoarthritis primarily affects the weight-bearing joints. It's easy to see how the burden of obesity aggravates the problem. The more pressure on the joint, the more painful it feels. The obvious solution is weight reduction, but it's not a simple thing to reduce the overweight elderly, especially those who are fairly inactive. The body is like a bank. If the calories taken in aren't spent, they accumulate. Weight reduction requires careful medical supervision and a high degree of motivation on the part of the person.

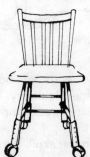

Chair with leg extenders for patients with arthritis. Courtesy of Campbell Soup Company.

    Osteoarthritis is treated with analgesics, physiotherapy, anti-inflammatory agents, and heat. The positioning of the body is important and a bed board and firm mattress are advised. Canes, cervical collars, and foot supports are often used. In cases of disabling pain and severely impaired function, the physician may suggest surgery. Reconstructive joint surgery and prostheses have helped many people to increase their mobility and obtain relief from pain.

2. *Rheumatoid Arthritis.* The cause of this disease of the connective tissue is unknown. Two or three times as many

women are affected by it as men. It has been seen in children as well as in the elderly. The symptoms are pain, heat, swelling in the joints and stiffness in the morning. The patient usually suffers muscle spasms, contractures, and enlarged joints of the wrists, hands, and feet. The joints' cartilage and ligaments are gradually destroyed.

The disease is treated systemically with corticosteroids, antiinflammatory agents, and analgesics. Local treatment consists of dry or moist heat, massage, optimum nutrition, and a program of adequate rest and exercise. Mechanical aids offer comfort. Some examples are canes, walkers, and a variety of self-help devices from chair leg extenders to specially designed kitchen utensils.

Certain surgical procedures, too, are designed to relieve the severe, disabling pain. Total joint replacement may offer relief in selected cases.

Both the patient and the patient's family need continuous emotional support as the disease is chronic and progressive, with exacerbations and remissions.

3. *Osteoporosis* is the result of demineralization of the bone. The chemical composition of the bone (calcium, phosphorus, etc.) doesn't change, but the amount of bone tissue diminishes so that the bones become less dense and more porous. This weakens them and they fracture easily. The long bones and the vertebral column are most vulnerable. This condition is found primarily in postmenopausal women; apparently there is a link between sex hormones and osteoporosis.

Another cause of osteoporosis is immobilization. When a patient is confined to bed for a long period of time, the calcium virtually leaches out of his bones.

Much of the distressing back pain endured by elderly persons is caused by compression fractures of the lower thoracic and lumbar vertebrae. These fractures can occur as a result of sneezing or of a coughing spell. In fact, back pain may be the reason a person visits a doctor and it may be then that the person first learns he has osteoporosis. Also associated with osteoporosis are postural changes such as kyphosis and a gradual loss of height. Most elderly people are well aware that they are a bit shorter at 70 than they were at 35.

4. *Contractures.* Because contractures develop quickly in the inactive older person, physical exercise is encouraged. Active exercise is best, of course, but if this is not possible, passive range-of-motion exercises should be given. If the person is ambulatory, his shoes should be well-fitted, as they are important to help provide a firm base of support and to help the patient keep a good sense of balance, especially on uneven surfaces. For both the ambulatory and nonambulatory patient, a corset or brace may be prescribed for comfort and support when sitting up.

5. *Accidents.* Many deaths over the age of 65 are the result of accidents, most frequently a fall. Any or all of the following elements for an accident may be present in an elderly person: diminished muscle strength, loss of hearing, poor eyesight, awkward gait, difficulty in maintaining balance, and a slow reaction when changing the position of the body. If the elderly adult doesn't understand the obvious hazards of the bathroom (hard, slippery surfaces, poorly labeled medications), the bedroom (scatter rugs, light cords), and the stairs, then someone responsible must assess the danger potential and eliminate it.

6. *Hip Fractures.* Elderly persons, particularly women, are prone to accidents that result in fractures of the hip. Curiously, the precipitating cause—usually a fall—is often insignificant, and makes one wonder which came first, the fall or the fracture.

The prognosis for those with hip fractures is much better today than it was 30 years ago. In fact, it was once regarded as a death sentence because of the long period of immobility it required. The aged patient who, with weakened physical defenses, was confined to bed, often developed a hypostatic pneumonia and died. Hypostatic pneumonia is still a very real threat, but with frequent turning, deep breathing exercises, range of motion exercises, and early ambulation, the risk is decidedly less. In addition, better infection control, improved nutrition, and physical therapy allow for a much more favorable outlook.

The treatment of a patient with a hip fracture usually begins with traction in order to prevent contractures, to relieve muscle spasm, and to prevent movement of bone fragments. A bed board is also used. The patient probably will be in a bed with a frame to which a trapeze has been attached to enable him to lift and move himself if possible.

When surgery is indicated, there are many types of pins, nails, and prostheses for the surgeon to choose from. The patient usually comes back from the operating room with a "wedge" type of support between the legs to maintain proper position. This device also helps when the patient is being turned from side to side. Standing, pivoting to sit in a chair, and walking with the aid of a walker usually follow.

7.   *Muscle Atrophy.* The loss of muscle mass in the elderly is the cause of diminished strength. There is actually a gradual decrease in the number of muscle fibers. Most elderly people have enough strength to do what they want to do within reason. Since the loss of muscle mass happens quite gradually over a long period of time, they make adaptations to compensate for it.

Safety rail for bathtub. Courtesy of Lumex, Inc.

8.   *Leg Cramps.* A common complaint of the elderly is that of severe leg cramps, usually in the calf, which most often occur at night. They may be caused by poor circulation or by fatigue, or by standing for long periods. They may also be

caused by the excessive use of diuretics, a frequent medication of the aged patient. The condition should be investigated medically.

Nursing Measures and Procedures

Patients in Traction

Traction means drawing or pulling. Traction is frequently used to pull the ends of broken bones, especially arm or leg bones, into proper alignment. In this way, the extremity may be immobilized and the bones kept in position for healing. Traction is also used in treating fractured vertebrae and for patients with muscle spasm.

Two kinds of traction are skin traction and skeletal traction. With skin traction, the force pulls on an extremity—a leg, for example—that has been prepared with adhesive or moleskin strips attached to a block positioned so there is no pressure on the side of the foot. The extremity is then wrapped in Ace or tensor bandages, whichever the physician orders. A rope is tied to the block, guided over a pulley, and fastened to a weight. With skeletal traction, the force is applied directly to a bone by means of pins or wires passed through the bone or by tongs (Crutchfield tongs are one type) anchored in the bone.

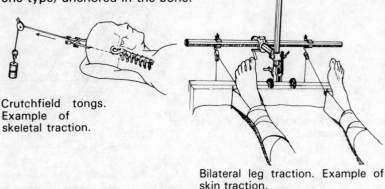

Crutchfield tongs.
Example of
skeletal traction.

Bilateral leg traction. Example of skin traction.

General Care of a Patient in Traction

1. see that the ropes are on the pulleys and are not frayed
2. see that the weights swing free of the bed and are not removed without a doctor's order

3. steady the weights when moving the bed
4. when a pillow is used to support the leg, check to see that there is no pressure on the heel or the back of the knee
5. inspect skin over all pressure points regularly
6. if skeletal traction is used, check for signs of infection around pin or wire site; cover sharp ends of pins with cork (guards) and be sure bed linen doesn't snag on pins or wires; change dressings PRN and use recommended skin care preparations
7. encourage patient to use tapeze to lift himself when using the bedpan or just to change his position, if only for a few seconds—even a few seconds off the pressure areas permit circulation of air to the skin
8. encourage patient to actively exercise all joints and muscles not affected by traction; include coughing and deep breathing
9. when making the occupied bed of a patient in traction, change the linen from top to bottom instead of from side to side
10. provide for comfort by use of toe socks if a foot is exposed, and inspect the bed covers to see that they don't interfere with traction
11. use foot support to prevent foot drop

NOTE: Avoid pressure at danger points and prevent rubbing of skin by edges of elastic wrapping bandages. Rubbing can cause erosion sores. Danger points are:

> any bony prominence—elbow, wrist, ankle, back of heel, spine, shoulder blades, iliac crest, sacral areas
>
> behind the knee where the peroneal nerve passes over the neck of the fibula
>
> the elbow where the ulnar nerve passes over the inner side

Additional information: Another application of traction is called "balanced suspension." This is suspending an extremity or other part of the body so it "floats" independently of the other parts of the body.

There are numerous types of traction and the preceding information is meant to acquaint the nurse with general information about traction. Each application of traction is done according to a specific physician's order. While two patients may have exactly the same fracture in exactly the same extremity, the chances are that their specific orders will be different. One doctor may allow his patient to be transported to x-ray out of traction and another will insist that traction is to be maintained at all times. Orders will have to be verified.

Patients with Total Hip and Knee Replacement

Total hip replacement is a surgical procedure used in treating several conditions including severe arthritis of the hip. It has provided dramatic relief from pain, correction of deformity, and increased mobility in selected cases.

The metal and plastic prosthesis is kept in place with screws or an intermedullary stem, or with an acrylic cement.

The operation carries considerable risk. The patients are usually elderly, quite a lot of blood is lost during surgery, and postoperatively there is the possibility of dislocation of the prosthesis, thromboembolic sepsis and infection. However, with careful nursing and medical management, the overall picture is optimistic and the procedure is being done with increasing frequency.

Total knee replacement is a surgical procedure that may give the patient with degenerative knee disease or rheumatoid knees marked relief from pain and improved knee motion.

The prosthesis is made of metal and plastic and is anchored in place with a plastic cement. Patients begin weight-bearing with a walker, then crutches, and gradually progress to a cane. In time, if it is comfortable, they may walk unaided.

Cast Care

A cast is applied in order to immobilize a part of the body and to permit early weight-bearing activities. It's usually made of plaster of Paris although there are some newer materials (fiberglass, for one) that are lightweight and can be wet. These, however, are quite expensive.

A cast that has just been applied should be exposed to the air so it dries, a process that takes about 48 hours. A dry cast is hard, white, and shiny.

Nursing care of the patient who has had a cast applied consists of reassuring him that the heat felt when the cast is newly applied is normal and that this heat occurs only while the cast is drying. This uncomfortable feeling is short-lived. Check skin color and movement and sensitivity of the parts of the limb not enclosed in the cast at stated intervals. Listen to the patient's complaints and report them! Pain, swelling, tingling, numbness, inability to move fingers or toes, blue fingernails or toenails must be reported immediately because these observations may indicate pressure on a nerve, constriction of blood vessels, or swelling of the part enclosed in the cast, which may lead to paralysis or tissue necrosis.

Sometimes casts have to be split (bivalved) if circulation is constricted. A physician determines what action to take based on the information elicited from the patient and the nurse.

Continuous emotional support is imperative. The elderly person already has diminished muscular strength and casts are heavy. Pain may also be present. Add to this the anticipation of a long period of rehabilitation or physiotherapy, and it is no wonder that patients in casts become depressed.

The foregoing instructions apply to the care of all patients in casts. The nurse will need to check physicians' orders as they apply to individual patients.

Positioning
A patient in bed may lie in three basic positions: on the back (dorsal), on the side (lateral), or on the abdomen (prone). Patients are sometimes put in variations of these three basic positions for various treatments and examinations. The nurse is responsible for knowing how to correctly position and drape the patient for examination and treatment.

Purposes
to prepare the patient for examination or treatment without
    unnecessary exposure
to provide comfort

Types of Positions

1. *Horizontal Recumbent Position (Supine).* Used for comfort and examination. Patient lies flat on back with legs together and extended (sometimes slightly flexed to relax abdominal muscles); pillow under head; arms at side of body.

2. *Dorsal Recumbent Position.* Used for vaginal and rectal examinations and treatments. Patient lies flat on back with knees flexed, draped with a sheet or bath blanket that is drawn back for the examination.

3. *Lithotomy Position.* Used for vaginal and rectal examinations. Same as dorsal recumbent except that the feet and legs are elevated about 18 inches above buttocks and the feet may be placed in stirrups.

4. *Prone Position.* Used for examination of back, spinal surgery, treatment of sacral decubitus ulcers. Patient lies on abdomen, head to the side, arms flexed beside head.

5. *Fowler's Position.* Used for comfort or when supine position is contraindicated. Head of the bed is elevated to a 45 degree angle. Variations: high Fowler's, low Fowler's.

6. *Sims' Position.* Used for rectal examination, enemas, inserting suppositories, taking rectal temperatures. Patient lies on left side with pillow under head, right knee flexed against the abdomen, left knee slightly flexed, left arm behind body, right arm beside head.

7. *Knee Chest Position (Genupectoral).* Used for rectal examination, vaginal exam, surgical procedures, and postpartum exercises. Patient on knees, chest on bed, arms in position of comfort, hips should be directly above knees, face to side.

8. *Trendelenberg Position.* Sometimes ordered for shock. Patient supine; head of bed is lower than foot so that the body is on an inclined plane slanting downward.

The position and arrangement of the parts of the body is called posture. Patients restricted to bed rest often have poor posture because they bend their backs while lying on their sides and flex their knees and hips. They may assume this position because they're cold or in pain. Good body alignment is a must for someone confined to bed for any length of time.

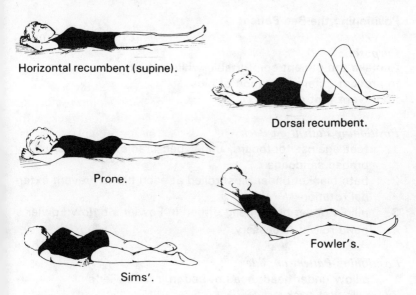

Horizontal recumbent (supine).

Dorsal recumbent.

Prone.

Fowler's.

Sims'.

POSITIONS.

A firm supporting mattress is the first requirement for achieving good body alignment. A frequent complication of bed rest is foot drop, which is an inability to bend the foot backward due to shortening of the gastrocnemius muscle. This can be prevented by not tucking the top linen in too tightly and by using a footboard against which the patient can place the soles of his feet. Be sure the footboard is covered with a linen protector. A bed cradle, a type of frame designed to keep covers off the feet, is also a helpful device. Good alignment of the feet may also be achieved by having the patient wear his shoes in bed, and some physicians approve of this. Since elderly people have poor circulation in their extremities, their feet are often cold. It's a good idea to keep the feet covered with socks or booties.

Other means of providing support for patients' position in bed are sandbags, pillows, rolled-up bath blankets, pads, or towels. When a patient is positioned on his side, a folded bath blanket should be placed between his knees, a pillow should be at his back, and another pillow should be under the uppermost arm.

Positioning the Bed Patient

Purposes
to make the patient comfortable while in bed
to prevent external rotation of hips
to prevent foot drop

Positioning Patient on Back
1. feet against footboard, under bed cradle, or supported by braced sandbags
2. bath blanket under hips, rolled at each hip to prevent external rotation
3. pillow under head; head of bed in Fowler's or low Fowler's
4. hand rolls if necessary

Positioning Patient on Side
1. pillow under head; head of bed in low Fowler's
2. pillow at back
3. top leg flexed, supported by pillow or folded bath blanket
4. arms in position of comfort
5. hand rolls if necessary

Positioning Patient Prone
(Verify with physician to determine if tolerable)
1. rolled bath blanket under ankles
2. head on small pillow, to one side
3. shoulder rolls or small pillow under abdomen if advisable
4. hand rolls

Restraints
Restraints are used for the protection of the patient and/or the safety of others. They are always ordered by the physician (except in cases of emergency) and should be used only as a last resort after all other attempts at calming the patient have failed.

Restraints must be used judiciously because they aggravate a person's fear, confusion, and hostility. What other approaches can the nurse take? First of all, reduce stimulation. If the environment is too noisy or crowded, the patient may have to be moved.

Sometimes massage relieves tension and anxiety. Speak quietly and distinctly. Frequently a patient responds better to one particular staff or family member. Testing some alternatives to restraints is an indication of sensitive nursing.

Purposes
to prevent the patient from injuring himself or others
to immobilize the patient temporarily (as for a treatment)
to provide support for the patient

Types of Restraints
1. Posey waist restraint—soft, belt model—limits movement—ties *under* bed or around chair
2. jacket restraint—limits movement but provides support—used in bed or chair
3. cloth wrist restraint—used to prevent patient from injuring himself by pulling out IVs, and so on
4. leg restraints—seldom used except under supervision
5. leather restraints—used in cases of severe hyperactivity and confusion

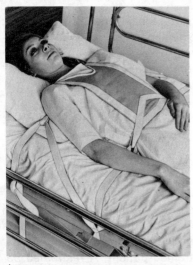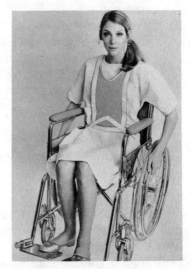

Restraints. Courtesy of Lumex, Inc.

Dangers of Restraints
1. may limit circulation
2. may cause skin breakdown
3. may contribute to such effects of immobility as: a) contractures; b) decubitus ulcers; c) hypostatic pneumonia; d) loss of muscle tone
4. may give staff members a false sense of security
5. may cause restrained patient to feel rage or to feel helpless

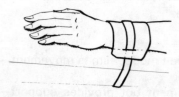 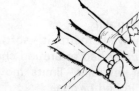

Hand restraint.

Leg or ankle restraint.

How to Avoid Restraint Dangers
1. check patient at regular intervals, removing and replacing restraints *one at a time* to look at the skin
2. keep skin under restraints clean and dry; apply lotion and massage
3. give range of motion exercises at least once on each shift; encourage active exercise when possible (i.e., walk with patients who can be ambulated)
4. relieve pressure on bony prominences
5. turn patients every two hours

   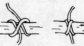

Single half hitch. Two half hitches. Clove hitch.

SAFETY TIES.

NOTE: Just because a patient is restrained does not mean that he needs less observation. The long cloth ties of restraints have built-in risks. Also, there always seems to be a "helpful" patient around who unties the restrained patient. *A restrained patient is vulnerable.*

Wheelchairs, Walkers, Canes, Crutches, Braces, and Prostheses

Wheelchairs. The infirmity of the patient should determine the type of wheelchair to be used. Some wheelchairs come with adjustable back rests, head rests, and leg and arm rests. Detachable swinging footrests may be either removed or swung out of the way to get closer to furniture or equipment. Hands that are weak or affected by arthritis can wheel a chair easier if knobs are provided on wheels. These projections transfer the work of the fingers to the palms of the hands. The brake should always be on when a patient is being moved in or out of a wheelchair.

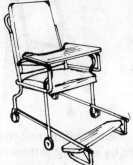

Multi-purpose wheelchair-table, often called a geri-chair. Used in hospitals and nursing homes for nonambulatory patients. The table provides passive restraint and table and chair give proper support for long term seating.

Wheelchair cushions are available from hospital supply firms; they help decrease the chances of pressure sores developing. Gel cushions filled with emulsions which shift with a patient's weight help to equalize pressure. A wheelchair should be kept clean and in good repair.

Walker. A walker is a light-weight metal frame with hand grips and safety-tipped legs. Some walkers have two front

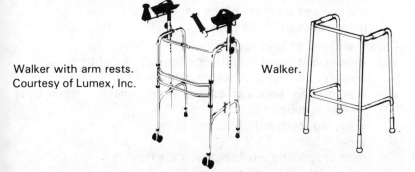

Walker with arm rests.   Walker.
Courtesy of Lumex, Inc.

wheels. The patient lifts or wheels the walker in front of him as he walks. Various carrier bags for walkers that are useful for holding small items are available.

Canes. Canes may be wood, metal, or plastic. A one-point cane has a curved handle and is used on the strong side of the body. There are also tripod and quad canes which stand alone. All

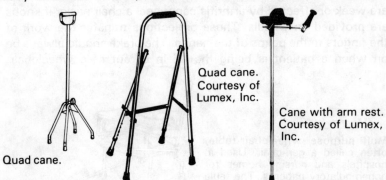

Quad cane.
Courtesy of
Lumex, Inc.

Cane with arm rest.
Courtesy of Lumex,
Inc.

Quad cane.

canes should have safety tips to prevent slipping. Patients should be measured by a physical therapist for canes and crutches. Often a safety belt is used by the one teaching a patient to walk (whether with cane, walker, or independently).

Crutches. Crutches are used after the patient has been measured either by the physician or by the physical therapist. The patient must have a broad base of support, that is, a well-fitted pair of shoes. Bedroom slippers are unsuitable. A patient's success with crutch walking depends on:

> the nature of the disability
> the age and strength of the patient
> the motivation of the patient

Crutch walking gaits include:

- 4-point gait (used if both legs can bear weight):
  right crutch, left foot, left crutch, right foot
- 3-point gait (requires strong arms because entire body weight is supported):
  weak leg, both crutches, strong leg
- 2-point gait:
  right crutch and left foot touch the floor
  left crutch and right foot touch the floor

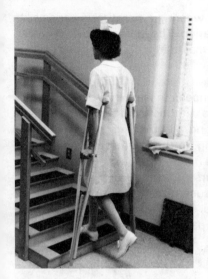
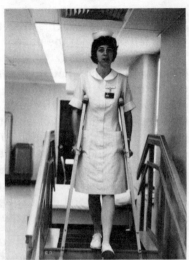

Ascending stairs: crutches on floor, foot on step. Feet before crutches.

Descending stairs: crutches go down a step ahead of feet.

- swinging-through gait (advanced):
  both legs lifted off ground, swing forward beyond crutches

NOTES: Lofstrand or forearm crutches eliminate axillary problems. Patients must be observed for weakness, fatigue, pallor, and diaphoresis. All ambulation aids should be kept close at hand so that they are there when needed.

Braces. Braces are supports for a part of the body with a musculoskeletal problem. They may immobilize, support, or protect, and are prescribed by a physician. Remember:
- braces should be cleaned and repaired when necessary
- check the condition of straps; look for missing or loose screws
- after removing the brace for bathing, check skin for any reddened areas

Prostheses. A prosthesis replaces a missing part of the body. For example, an artificial breast is used for a patient who has had a mastectomy. A patient who has had an amputation will be fitted with a prosthesis and trained in its use. The length of time a patient needs to master the art of wearing a prosthesis varies with his condition and with his motivation. The main purpose of an artificial leg is to help the patient maintain mobility.

Lifting and Moving Patients

One of the first things the nurse needs to learn in order to practice effective nursing is to assess a situation before taking action. When the situation involves lifting and moving, it's essential to size up the load before beginning. In the interest of comfort and safety for the patient *and for the nurse,* the practice of good body mechanics takes priority. The nurse who impulsively tries to lift or move an excessive load because time is short or because everyone else is too busy to help, is one who eventually will have an accident involving either the patient or herself. Or both.

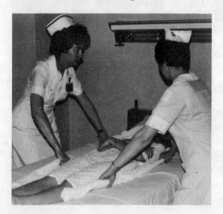

Using a turning sheet to lift a helpless patient. Note that the nurses' hips and knees are flexed.

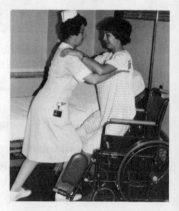

For safety's sake, the wheelchair is locked before nurse gets patient into it .

Purposes

to lift and move patients and objects safely and comfortably
to protect one's self and one's patients by practicing the principles
    of good body mechanics

Basic Principles of Body Mechanics

1.   center of gravity—concentration of weight of the body on
       point around which all parts of the body balance each other

(in a standing position, this brings the center of gravity inside
the pelvis slightly anterior to the upper part of the sacrum)
2.   line of balance—imagine a vertical line through the center of
the body (remember this when using your stronger muscles)
3.   base of support (feet)—center of gravity is over base of support

Directions for Lifting and Moving
1.   assess situation: if you will need help, get it
2.   encourage patient to help himself as much as possible
3.   keep your back erect
4.   stand with your feet apart
5.   stand close to object to be moved
6.   flex your knees and hips
7.   carry things close to your body
8.   roll or turn patient or object instead of lifting, if possible
9.   use a turning sheet under a helpless patient to pull him up in
bed
10. raise or lower bed until its height is comfortable to work at
before lifting or moving patient

Range of Motion (ROM)
"Use it or lose it!"

Flexibility and muscle tone are soon lost without exercise.
Range of motion exercises should be carried out on all patients
confined to bed at least once each day unless specifically contraindicated by the physician. For many, it may be their only exercise.

These exercises are done to prevent contractures, improve
circulation, maintain joint mobility, and in general induce a feeling
of well-being. The exercises must be planned to use the muscles
necessary to maintain joint mobility. The structure of a joint limits
its movement; for example, hinge joints don't rotate but move in
one direction only. Ideally, each joint should be put through its
full range of movement daily. This is why patients should be encouraged to do as much of their own care as possible. It helps
keep the joints flexible and the muscles toned. Besides, the independence is good psychologically.

But what if the range of motion exercises can't be done actively by the patient? Then the nurse, or whoever is giving the bedside care, should give ROM passively. A good time to carry out ROM exercises is during the bed bath. Enlist the cooperation of patients by telling them why ROM exercises are essential and just what will be done.

Exercising should not be done when the patient is tired or in pain.

The following are suggested range of motion exercises.

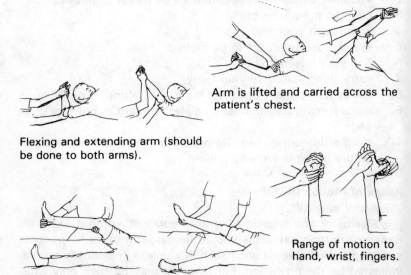

Arm is lifted and carried across the patient's chest.

Flexing and extending arm (should be done to both arms).

Range of motion to hand, wrist, fingers.

Flexion and extension of legs.

REVIEW

A. Multiple Choice (Select the Best Answer)

1. Involuntary muscles:
    1. accumulate lactic acide as waste
    2. work automatically
    3. are made up of striated muscle fibers
    4. are attached to bones

2. Joints are also called:
   1. articulations
   2. cancellous
   3. hyoid
   4. fibrous
3. Adhesions that form between cartilages cause:
   1. bleeding
   2. pallor
   3. overgrowth of bone
   4. impaired function
4. Osteoarthritis is:
   1. a disease of connective tissue
   2. degenerative joint disease
   3. cured by aspirin
   4. most common in men
5. Osteoporosis is:
   1. caused by immobilization
   2. confined to postmenopausal women
   3. another term for osteoarthritis
   4. cured by increased calcium intake

B. Matching Test (Match Column 1 with Column 2)

Column 1	Column 2
a. gastrocnemius	_____6. heel
b. traction	_____7. drawing or pulling
c. Achilles tendon (location)	_____8. behind the knee
d. peroneal nerve (location)	_____9. calf muscle
e. lateral	_____10. side

C. Briefly Answer the Following Questions

1. Give three rules for the general care of a patient in traction.
2. Why are elderly people often prone to accidents?
3. Name one cause of the distressing back pain endured by many elderly.
4. What should the nurse check for in observing her patient who has just had a cast put on?
5. What are the dangers of restraints?

12

The Circulatory System

Objectives

After completing this chapter, the student should be able to:

- better understand how aging affects the circulatory system
- help the congestive heart failure patient get his disease under control
- do the procedures for soaks, foot care, and stump care
- take vital signs
- apply elasticized stockings and bandages
- know the nursing responsibilities for anticoagulant therapy
- use the following words correctly

Vocabulary

The following words relate to the material in this chapter. Look up the ones that you do not know or are not sure of.

apical	Cheyne-Stokes	stasis
apnea	edema	stertorous
brachial artery	popliteal artery	varicose
carotid artery	rales	ventricle

Anatomy Review

The blood is a vital fluid that keeps flowing along, distributing oxygen and food to all parts of the body while removing carbon dioxide, a waste product. It is kept moving by the continuous pumping action of the heart.

Other Functions

The blood also helps fight infection through the action (phagocytosis) of the white blood cells, and just by its circulation it helps to maintain our body temperature. For example, if we are too warm, the capillaries of the skin expand, more blood flows through them, and the increased blood volume allows for a greater heat exchange. This results in a lower body temperature.

When there is external trauma to a blood vessel, we observe another characteristic of blood. It clots. Normally, blood is a liquid that flows smoothly through our blood vessels. But if a vessel is damaged, blood cells called platelets plug it up and then start releasing certain substances that produce a clot. Eventually this forms a scab.

When there is trauma to a blood vessel which causes its inner smooth lining to become rough, the same thing happens. In the aged, arteriosclerosis causes the inner lining of the arteries to become thickened and rough, and this encourages clot formation.

Structures

Blood Vessels. Arteries, veins, and capillaries are the three types of blood vessels. Arteries carry blood *from* the heart toward capillaries in the body's tissues. Veins carry blood away from capillaries *toward* the heart. A capillary is the body's smallest blood vessel and it's just wide enough for a red blood cell to pass through. Capillaries are microscopic in size. In a schematic drawing they appear as a web of fine tubules that branch out from arteries and unite with venules (small veins). Thus the vessels form a closed system by which the blood circulates throughout the body.

An arterial wall is tough and heavy, built to withstand a lot of pressure. The largest artery is the aorta. A vein is much thinner because the pressure of the blood within it is less. The largest vein is the vena cava.

Heart.   The heart is a powerful, cone-shaped, hollow muscle. This tireless, fist-sized organ beats over 100,000 times a day to supply blood to over 100,000 miles of blood vessels in the body.

Inside the heart is a septum (partition) that divides it in half. The four chambers of the heart are the right and left atria and right and left ventricles. There also are valves that make sure the blood flows in the right direction. The tricuspid (three-pointed) valve is between the right atrium and the right ventricle; the mitral valve is between the left atrium and left ventricle. Semilunar valves monitor the blood flowing from the ventricles to the arteries.

Each side of the heart has its own job. The right side takes blood that is loaded with carbon dioxide, a waste product, and pumps in *to* the lungs. There, the waste is removed and oxygen is added. Then the left side of the heart receives the blood *from* the lungs and sends it throughout the body.

Age-Related Changes

1. *Arteriosclerosis.*   The most common type of vascular change that occurs in the aged is the development of arteriosclerosis, a condition marked by a loss of elasticity and associated narrowing of the walls of the blood vessels, particularly the arteries. Arteriosclerosis is sometimes referred to as atherosclerosis; the words are often used interchangeably. Plaque, deposits of fat and sometimes of calcium, builds up inside the arterial walls. We're not certain

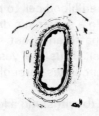

Lumen of normal artery.

Narrowed lumen due to arteriosclerotic changes in blood vessel.

why this happens. It may be caused by one's diet, the stress of disease, hereditary factors, or the process of aging.

The effects of arteriosclerosis are diverse. Systemically, it may result in an insufficient supply of blood to the cells of certain organs with the consequence that the cells die. Vital organs which can be affected are the brain, the heart, and the kidneys.

A local effect can also cause clotting problems. A healthy blood vessel collapses when it is cut, thereby encouraging clotting. Thickened arteries can't collapse readily, so bleeding continues. That's why hemorrhage is a real threat to the elderly surgical patient. Perversely, the deposition of plaque on the blood vessel lining encourages clots to form and this is dangerous. These clots can occlude an artery, causing severe pain, necrosis, and ultimately, death.

2. *Vascular Degeneration.* Good health practices can prevent, or at least alleviate, the problems of vascular degeneration. Neglected foot infections and varicose ulcers are commonly seen on the routine hospital admission of elderly patients. While heredity plays a part in the role of varicose veins, obesity, and poor posture (standing for long hours without a change of position or elevating the legs) increase the destructive process. Leg ulcers frequently occur in the elderly who have diabetes and these lesions require prompt medical treatment. Nutritional adjustments, medications, warm compresses, and rest are utilized to bring relief.

3. *Amputations.* When vascular problems do not respond to conservative treatment, an elderly patient may be faced with amputation. The shock is severe and demands not only the patient's physical care but also supportive emotional care. The nurse's attitude needs to be positive because the patient fears that if he loses one foot or leg, it will be only a matter of time before he loses the other. Postoperatively, independence and self-care should be encouraged as well as specific exercises designed to strengthen muscles and prevent flexion contractures.

4. *Aneurysms.* In the elderly, aneurysms usually occur in patients who have marked arteriosclerosis. An aneurysm is a

balloonig out of a wall of an artery. The symptoms are severe pain, profound weakness, and shock. In this acute condition, surgery is the usual treatment.

5. *Heart Size.* The size of the heart does not change in the elderly as a rule. An enlarged heart indicates some heart disease, but it's not due just to aging. The resting heart rate doesn't change much with age either. But maximum heart rate decreases with age. For example, a 20-year-old can, through exercise, increase his heart rate to over 200 beats per minute. The average exercising 80-year-old has a maximum heart rate of 120-130 beats per minute.

6. *Reduced Cardiac Output.* In the elderly, each heartbeat puts out less blood volume than in younger persons. Reduced cardiac output and low maximum heart rate limit the amount of blood that flows to the various parts of the body. This explains why elderly people tire more easily than younger people. However, prudent exercise can increase endurance in the aged. Walking is the best exercise.

7. *Hypertension.* Hypertension is a natural accompaniment to arteriosclerosis. As the lumen of the vessel narrows, the heart has to work harder pumping blood. High blood pressure can cause heart failure, kidney failure, or stroke. (see Chapter 14).

8. *Congestive Heart Failure* (CHR). In congestive heart failure there is diminished cardiac output, which means that food and oxygen no longer get to vital organs as needed. When the blood supply to the kidney is insufficient, there is a problem with filtrating sodium. The patient tends to retain water, as is evidenced by the puffy, edematous legs of these people. The blood coming from veins and capillaries *toward* the heart backs up and congestion ensues. This contributes to dependent edema.

9. *Pulmonary edema* is severe congestion of the lungs that occurs with congestive heart failure. Not enough blood leaves the lungs from the *left* side of the heart and the blood keeps getting into the lungs from the *right* side. Fluid collects in the alveoli and the blood in the capillaries doesn't gather enough oxygen. The patient appears dyspneic, cyanotic, and anxious.

He has a rapid pulse and low blood pressure. He coughs continually and may even spit up blood. An emergency situation exists because he can actually drown in his own secretions.

Nursing Measures and Procedures

Helping the CHF Patient Cope
Congestive heart failure can be controlled, but the patient must be educated and motivated to follow a therapeutic program. The nurse may help by:
1. emphasizing the importance of taking prescribed medications *exactly* as ordered
2. seeing that the patient understands and carries out his low sodium diet instructions
3. stressing the importance of adhering *strictly* to his diet
4. suggesting daily weighing at the *same time each day* to check for fluid retention
5. explaining the importance of rest and exercise
6. teaching the danger signs of recurrent pathology: weight gain; anorexia; shortness of breath; coughing; and swelling of feet, legs, ankles (the patient should be urged to communicate *any* of these symptoms to his physician immediately)

Soaks
Warm soaks to the extremities are ordered to increase circulation, encourage healing, relax tissue, and inhibit infection. After soaking, medication may be applied. Soaks are a useful therapy but they must be used with caution at all times, particularly when the patient is elderly. Many aged patients have peripheral circulatory problems and are vulnerable to heat injury. Their reflexes are slower and this interferes with their response to pain.

It isn't practical to give a definite temperature and length of time for soaks. These judgments depend on the condition of the patient, the quality of the skin on the part to be soaked, and the size of the area to be soaked. Generally, most soaks involve putting an extremity into a prescribed solution for a given period of time. If it's an open wound, a sterile foot tub is obtained from central supply, and dressings are applied as needed after the soak.

When a warm compress is ordered *to be applied continually,* the nurse uses an electric heating device designed to keep wet dressings warm at a constant temperature for an extended period of time. The usual safety precautions that apply to electrical devices are employed: checking wiring and plugs, avoiding the use of safety pins around the heating element, and, above all, emphasizing the *responsibility* of the patient to report any discomfort or overheating.

Foot Care

The geriatric patient often has foot problems that may be related to peripheral vascular disease. Good foot care can result in the patient's increased mobility. At the very least, it can prevent complications in patients who have diabetes and circulatory problems that affect the extremities.

Purposes
to improve circulation of the lower extremities
to prevent infection
to provide comfort
to promote cleanliness

Equipment

basin	mild soap	nail clippers
soft cloth and towel	lotion	emery board

Sequence
1. soak feet in lukewarm water
2. check skin surfaces for signs of infection, blisters, peeling, lesions
3. wash with mild soap, soft cloth
4. rinse
5. dry thoroughly and gently with soft towel, especially between the toes
6. trim nails with toenail clippers; smooth with emery board; *if nails are thick and long, a podiatrist should be employed*
7. apply lotion or cream before putting on clean socks or stockings

NOTE: A daily foot soak and a daily change of socks and stockings that fit well is important. Self-care with over-the-counter liquids that dissolve corns and calluses should be discouraged. They can be destructive to sensitive tissues. The elderly should also avoid using razor blades and pointed scissors for their foot care. Shoes should be well-constructed to give support and should be well-fitted for comfort.

Taking Vital Signs

Vital signs, sometimes called cardinal symptoms, are those which can be measured. They are taken to help monitor a patient's condition. Strictly speaking, blood pressure and pulse (its rate and character) are the vital signs that belong with the circulatory system. However, procedures for taking respirations and temperature will be included in this section because these data are often obtained at the same time.

When an artery expands and contracts, the throbbing (pulse) that can be felt in an artery near the surface of the body is the blood being forced through the vessel by the beating of the heart. We usually time the pulse by locating the radial artery at the wrist. At times we take an apical pulse by counting the heartbeats with a stethoscope. (Other arteries where the pulse can be felt include the carotid, temporal, brachial, femoral, and popliteal arteries.)

Taking a radial pulse.

Sequence for Taking Pulse (Radial)

1. identify patient; explain procedure
2. position patient's arm comfortably across his chest
3. place your first three or four fingers on the palm side of the patient's wrist close to the thumb (do not use *your* thumb; it has a pulse of its own)
4. time the pulse for one full minute using second hand of watch
5. note the character of the pulse—whether strong, weak, regular, irregular, bounding, and so on
6. document on graphic sheet as per institution's policy

Sequence for Taking Pulse (Apical)

1. using a stethoscope, listen for heartbeat to left of sternum
2. count heartbeat for one full minute by second hand of watch
3. document appropriately on a graphic sheet

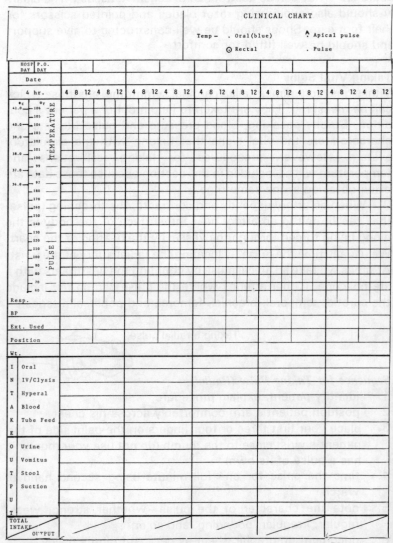

Example of a graphic sheet. Courtesy of Baystate Medical Center

NOTE: Unusually rapid heartbeat (pulse) is called tachycardia; unusually slow heartbeat is called bradycardia. These are significant observations and must be reported immediately. Pulse rhythm may be regular or irregular. Descriptions of any irregularity must be documented and reported.

Respirations

Respirations should be counted when the patient is unaware of the procedure. This can be done at the time the pulse is being taken, when the patient has his arm across his chest. If someone knows his breathing rate is being timed, he may subconsciously alter it. The rate and character of respirations is noted to show either the progress or the change in a patient's condition.

One inhalation and one exhalation is counted as a respiration. A normal adult rate is about 16 per minute. Respirations are also described as shallow, labored, or difficult. If they fall into any of these categories, the patient's color should also be observed and the findings documented and reported.

Sequence for Taking Respirations

1. while taking pulse with patient's arm across chest, prepare to count respirations
2. observe each rise and fall of the chest and count as one respiration
3. time for one full minute
4. document as per hospital policy recording rate, depth, and any unusual characteristics

Blood Pressure

Blood pressure is the force that the blood exerts against the walls of the arteries as it is being pumped through the body by the heart. The equipment used to measure it is a stethoscope and a blood pressure cuff (sphygmomanometer). There are two types of cuffs: a *mercury* sphygmomanometer has numbers on the glass column that contain the mercury and the *aneroid* type has numbers on a dial that are read as the blood pressure is heard.

The reading obtained when the first sound is read measures the pressure of the blood at the height of the contraction phase of the heartbeat, which is called the systole. The reading at the last sound heard is a register of the blood pressure at the resting phase of the heart, called the diastole.

Arteries that have lost elasticity cause pressure to be high. Other factors responsible for high blood pressure are exercise, stimulants, and excitement. Average adult pressure is 120 for systolic pressure and 80 for diastolic pressure (120/80), although these figures rise with age. A pressure of (150/90) might be considered normal for a person 70 years old. Generally, systolic pressures over 150 are considered high and diastolic pressures over 90 are also considered high. Low blood pressure in healthy adults is rarely significant (90 to 105 systolic). To take blood pressures:

1. identify patient, explain procedure
2. patient's arm at the level of the heart
3. wrap cuff around patient's bare arm
4. locate brachial artery by palpation; place stethoscope over artery
5. inflate cuff while listening to pulsations
6. inflate cuff 20 points above that at which the pulse is no longer heard
7. slowly deflate cuff reading the *first* figure heard; the reading at this point is the systolic pressure
8. continue deflating cuff until *no* sound is heard; the reading at this point is diastolic pressure
9. document as per hospital policy; report abnormal readings immediately

NOTE: Unless you use your own stethoscope continually, remember to clean off the earpieces of the available stethoscope with an alcohol wipe.

Temperatures
Body temperature is the balance between the body's heat production and heat loss. Heat is generated by the metabolism of food. Exercise, external application of heat, and infection also cause an increase in body temperature. Heat is normally lost through perspiration and respiration. Hemorrhage and starvation also cause loss of body heat.

Two types of thermometers are used for registering body temperature—one based on the Fahrenheit scale and one based on the centigrade (or Celsius) scale. The Fahrenheit thermometer is most commonly used in health care facilities in this country. Body temperature is most often taken by placing a thermometer under the tongue for three minutes, but in certain circumstances it can be taken by placing the thermometer in the rectum for three minutes or in the axilla for ten minutes.

Some health facilities use electronic thermometers. The thermometer probe is covered with a disposable plastic probe cover and is inserted into the patient's mouth or rectum. The temperature is read on a small screen.

Normal oral adult body temperature is 98.6°F; rectal temperature reading is usually one degree *higher* and an axillary temperature is usually one degree *lower* than an oral temperature.

Oral temperature must not be taken on:
1.   very young children (five years or under)
2.   unconscious or confused patients
3.   patients who have had oral surgery
4.   certain patients on oxygen therapy
5.   *any* patient with a condition where the nurse deems it inadvisable to take the temperature orally.

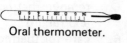
Oral thermometer.

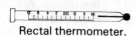
Rectal thermometer.

Oral Temperatures
1.   identify patient, explain procedure
2.   check thermometer for possible defects (mercury that doesn't shake down, illegible markings, cracks, etc.)

To convert centigrade to Fahrenheit, multiply by 9/5 and add 32. To change Fahrenheit to centigrade, subtract 32 and multiply by 5/9.

Examples of Equivalents

Centigrade	Fahrenheit
37.0	98.6
37.5	99.5
38.0	100.4
38.5	101.3
39.0	102.2
40.0	104.0
41.0	105.8

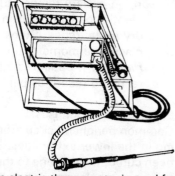
An electric thermometer is used for oral, rectal, and axillary temperatures.

3. shake thermometer until mercury registers 96°F or below
4. place under patient's tongue; tell patient *not* to bite down; tell patient to keep in place in *closed* mouth for three minutes
5. remove thermometer, clean off, read; jot down reading in notebook
6. care for thermometer as per facility's policy
7. document temperature reading; report abnormalities immediately

Rectal Temperatures

1. identify patient, explain procedure, screen patient
2. lubricate end of rectal thermometer (after steps 2 and 3 above)
3. place patient in lateral position
4. insert thermometer 1½'' and *hold* it for three minutes
5. remove thermometer after three minutes; wipe clean; read and record
6. care for thermometer as per facility's policy
7. document reading, report temperature of over 100°F immediately

NOTE: Rectal temperatures are contraindicated in cases of rectal surgery or rectal inflammations.

Axillary Temperatures

If both oral and rectal temperatures are contraindicated for any reason, an axillary temperature may be taken
1. identify patient, explain procedure
2. dry axilla; repeat Steps 2 and 3 of ORAL TEMPERATURE
3. place thermometer in axilla for 10 minutes; *hold thermometer* if patient is unable to cooperate
4. read and record as per facility's policy

Elasticized Stockings

Common peripheral circulatory problems cause edema and swelling in the lower extremities. Even after an attack of phlebitis has been cured, the damage to the valves in the vein may be such that they can no longer prevent backflow. This results in chronic venostasis, swelling, edema, and eventually, leg ulcers. Elasticized stockings are useful in the conservative management of this condition. These stockings help to prevent backflow of blood in the lower extremities. They must be correctly fitted so as to exert uniformly decreasing pressure from the foot upward. The stockings may be ordered in two lengths; foot to below the knee and foot to thigh.

Sequence

1. identify and screen patient; explain procedure
2. check to be sure legs and feet are clean and dry. If there is an ulceration, be sure that the dressing is dry and intact
3. lightly powder the foot to decrease friction
4. roll stocking; stretch and ease over toes, gradually unrolling as foot and leg is covered
5. check toes for motion and sensitivity after stockings are on

NOTE: These stockings should be changed daily. If the patient is confined to bed, the feet and legs should be bathed at least daily and the stockings removed and *reapplied* twice a day.

Elasticized Bandages

Ace or tensor bandages are made of woven elastic and covered with another fiber. They are used to support or immobilize an extremity, to apply pressure to a part of the body, to hold a bulky

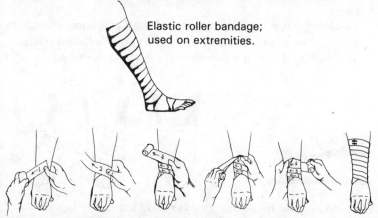

Elastic roller bandage; used on extremities.

Putting on an elastic bandage.

dressing in place, or if the patient has a skin reaction to tape of any kind.

An Ace bandage should be applied firmly enough to keep it in place but not so tightly that it interferes with circulation. When used on an extremity, the arm or leg should be observed at regular intervals for color, motion, and sensitivity.

Elasticized bandages come in a wide variety of widths and lengths. They are used only by a physician's order.

Stump Bandaging, Stump Care

As with all surgery, postoperative orders vary with the individual. Generally, early ambulation is encouraged. Casts are often used and patients may be able to use a prosthesis after 24 hours. An elderly patient needs special care because he may be dazed by the surgery and may not appear to know what type of surgery was performed even though he knew before the operation. Postoperative care includes:

1. observation for shock and hemorrhage (tourniquet to be kept at bedside stand)
2. use of stump sock to help shrink and shape stump to prosthesis
3. use of elasticized bandage with or without stump sock
4. encouraging patient to turn from side to side and to assume prone position if possible to help prevent flexion contractures
5. elevating lower part of bed rather than elevating stump on pillow. The stump should *not* be held up in a flexed position as this might cause a permanent flexion deformity.

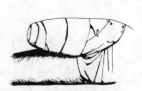
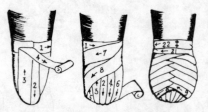
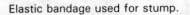

Elastic bandage used for stump.   Example of stump bandaging.

What the Nurse Should Know About Anticoagulant Therapy

Placing a patient on a medication that delays the clotting time of the blood and prevents further clot formation is referred to as anticoagulant therapy. It is prescribed for patients with the following problems.

thrombophlebitis
recurrent clot formation
congestive heart failure
hip fractures that may immobilize elderly patient for a long time

This therapy is not without risk and some physicians feel that the risks outweigh the gains. The primary complication is bleeding from or into any part of the body. Some examples are: bruises caused by trauma to tissues; bleeding from minor cuts such as shaving nicks; bleeding from the nose; bleeding from the gums; bleeding from IV sites; and bleeding from the urinary or gastrointestinal tracts.

Anticoagulants

Heparin Sodrium Derivatives (parenterally administered)	Coumarin Derivatives (administered orally)
Hepathrom	Dicumarol
Lipo-Hepin	Coumadin

Nursing Responsibilities
1. warn patient not to take *any* other medication without the physician's knowledge
2. tell patient to inform other health care professionals (dentists, podiatrists) that he's on anticoagulants
3. advise wearing of Medic-alert bracelet
4. emphasize the importance of the prescribed laboratory tests (prothrombin time, clotting time) that will be ordered on an out-patient basis
5. inspect the skin for bruises
6. report any bleeding from nose, mouth, or gums
7. observe urine for any signs of blood

NOTE: When administering anticoagulants to hospitalized patients, the nurse must verify the *most recent* laboratory values first.

REVIEW

A. Multiple Choice (Select the Best Answer)

1. The blood, a vital fluid, removes wastes. An example of a waste product is:
   a. oxygen
   b. carbon dioxide
   c. capillary
   d. venule
2. "Arteriosclerosis" is often called:
   a. atherosclerosis
   b. scoliosis
   c. varicose veins
   d. aneurysms
3. The rales heard in the pulmonary edema of congestive heart failure are due to:
   a. pneumonia
   b. hemoptysis
   c. anorexia
   d. fluid in alveoli
4. The patient with congestive heart failure should immediately report:
   a. shortness of breath
   b. drowsiness
   c. pruritus
   d. anxiety
5. Elderly patients receiving soaks are vulnerable to:
   a. jaundice
   b. dyspnea
   c. heat injury
   d. diaphoresis

B. Matching Test (Match Column 1 with Column 2)

Column 1   *Column 2*

a. vital sign   —— 6. first blood pressure sound
                                             heard
b. apical pulse   —— 7. noisy breathing
c. stertorous   —— 8. is heard left of sternum
d. systole   —— 9. resting phase of heart
e. diastole   ——10. blood pressure

C.   Briefly Answer the Following Questions

1. List three danger signs of recurrent congestive heart failure.
2. In what circumstances would oral temperatures be contraindicated?
3. Why shouldn't a pillow be used to elevate a stump?
4. Name one nursing responsibility in anticoagulant therapy.

13

The Genitourinary System

Objectives

Upon completing this chapter, the student should be able to:
- better understand how aging affects the genitourinary system
- do the procedures for catheterization, douche, Foley catheter irrigation, and obtaining a clean catch urine specimen
- assist with the pelvic examination
- record intake and output
- induce patients to void
- assist patients with bladder training
- use the following words correctly

Vocabulary

The following words relate to the material in this chapter. Look up the ones you do not know or are not sure about.

acid base balance	hypertrophy	pathogen
dyspareunia	myasthenia gravis	prophylaxis
escherichia coli	nocturia	pyelonephritis
frequency	Papanicolaou smear	sphincter
glomerulus	parenteral	turgor

Anatomy Review

Structures and Functions

Kidneys. The kidneys, two bean-shaped organs that lie just below the diaphragm on the posterior abdominal wall on either side of the spine and behind the peritoneum, are very important organs of excretion. Blood reaches the kidneys by way of the renal arteries and wastes are strained from the blood as it passes through the kidneys.

Nephrons. Nephrons are the kidneys' filtering units and there are millions of them screening out substances not needed by the body. Nephrons accept certain substances from the blood, and these substances are reabsorbed into the body. They also regulate water and electrolyte balance. The body has tremendous reserves and we are constructed so we can lose vast amounts of nephrons to age and disease and still live. In fact, we can lose a kidney, one-half of the filtering "team," and live normally.

Urine. Urine is the end product of the primary functions of the nephrons. It consists of filtered waste substances, excess salts, and water. Certain conditions of the urine mean that disease is present. For example, sugar in the urine (glycosuria) is a symptom of diabetes mellitus. Copious, dilute urine (polyuria) is a symptom of diabetes insipidus. Pus in the urine (pyuria) indicates an infection in the urinary system.

Ureters. The body has two ureters. They are tubes, each about 25 cm (ten inches) long, that extend from the renal pelvis (the kidney interior) to the bladder. Urine is passed from the kidneys into the ureters and then propelled by peristalsis down the ureters until it pools in the bladder.

Urethra. The urethra is also a tube, but thicker than the ureter. It extends from the bladder to the exterior. In the male, the urethra is about eight inches long because it runs through the penis. In the female, it is about one- and a-half inches long. Urine doesn't drip right through the bladder and urethra to the outside because a sphincter controls the meatus, which is the opening at the end of the urethra through which urine passes out of the body. The bladder relaxes and expands as the urine begins to fill it. As it fills to a certain level, contractions are triggered which force the fluid to exert pressure against the base of the urethra and the sphincter muscle. This we interpret as the desire to urinate.

Age-Related Changes

1. *Loss of Nephrons.* With aging, the kidneys function less efficiently. The number of nephrons decreases. A newborn has about a million nephrons in each kidney. A 75-year-old has about half of that number. The nephron, which filters the blood, also regulates the acid base balance in blood plasma. This is important to know when giving medications to the elderly because of the lesser number of nephrons in the older person's body. Thus, an elderly patient may exhibit an undesirable reaction to an average adult dosage of a drug.

2. *Arteriosclerotic Changes.* Arteriosclerosis may affect the blood vessels that supply blood to the urinary system. The reduction in the amount of blood going to the kidneys lowers their ability to resist infection and to recover from trauma.

3. *Reduced Muscle Tone of Genitourinary Organs.* The bladder, ureters, and urethra become less elastic with age and have poorer muscle tone. The capacity of the bladder often diminishes by half, and the urge to urinate doesn't occur until that capacity is nearly reached. As a consequence, many elderly are troubled by frequency, urgency, and nocturia. It's

easy to see how, in an institutional setting where an elderly patient is on medication and confined to bed, incontinence develops.

4. *Prostatic Enlargement.* In elderly males a common problem is enlargement of the prostate gland which surrounds the urethra. Symptoms of benign prostatic hypertrophy are nocturia, difficulty in starting to urinate, and narrowing of the stream (because of the obstruction). The treatment is prostatectomy.

5. *Calculi.* Residual urine is often associated with the development of calculi. If an elderly patient is immobilized, for example, with a fractured hip, the chance of developing calculi increases. While the cause of stone formation isn't completely understood, we do know that with failure to excrete certain substances (uric acid, calcium phosphate) stones may form.

6. *Glomerulonephritis.* Glomerulonephritis is present in many aged patients who do not have any obvious symptoms. It frequently isn't discovered until there's a noticeable elevation of blood pressure or swelling of the extremities. Stroke can trigger glomerulonephritis. Beginning symptoms are polyuria, nocturia, and frequency. In severe cases the body becomes "waterlogged" with fluid collecting in the chest cavity, the abdominal cavity (ascites), and the sac that encloses the heart. Unchecked, the patient slips into uremia.

7. *Urinary Tract Infections.* Escherichia coli is a bacterium that is a normal inhabitant of the human intestinal tract. It is frequently a cause of infections in the urinary tract. Hospital employees who do not practice good personal hygiene may carry this organism on their hands and so infect either themselves or their patients. Other bacteria can cause such infections. Obviously, the elderly patient is especially vulnerable either because of being confined to bed or because he has an indwelling Foley catheter. Ambulatory elderly patients may develop urinary tract infections if they don't use proper hygienic measures after urinating or after a bowel movement. Nurses should see that these patients wash their hands before meals and after using the bathroom. Nurses themselves must do the same and, in addition, they must wash their hands after handling drainage tubing or

bags and before giving direct patient care. Good nursing care includes encouraging fluids, observing and reporting temperature elevations and foul smelling urine, and giving special care to the external urinary meatus of any patient with an indwelling Foley catheter by washing the genitals when giving the daily bath and applying a topical antibiotic to help prevent infection.

a.   *Pyelonephritis* is a serious urinary tract infection often seen concurrently with another infection. For example, a patient who has an oral infection may develop a kidney infection. Any one of many pathogenic bacteria may cause pyelonephritis.

If the passage of urine from the kidney to the bladder is slowed down for any reason, an infection such as pyelonephritis can ensue. Particular attention must be paid to a patient who has an obstruction anywhere in the urinary tract or who has urinary stasis because the microorganisms migrate upward. Likely candidates are those who are immobilized for a long period of time. Meticulous catheter care of the patients who have indwelling (Foley) catheters and handwashing after touching *any* such patient with a catheter are essential. Health care personnel must wash hands when going from patient to patient because the microorganisms that thrive in the drainage bags are extremely resistant to antibiotics.

b.   *Cystitis* is an inflammation of the urinary bladder. Pathogens migrate from the kidneys downward or from the urethra up to the bladder. There are numerous other causes: enlarged prostate, urethral stricture, kidney infection, and, in women, improper perineal hygiene. Also, as mentioned earlier, the bladder loses muscle tone over the years. In fact, some bladders actually develop diverticuli, i.e., they become floppy with pockets that trap urine. When this residual urine becomes infected, cystitis results. While an elderly person may put off seeking medical help for many infirmities, they usually consult a physician for cystitis because of the painful urination that accompanies this infection.

Women have a much higher incidence of cystitis than men because of their short urethra and the location of the meatus, which is easily contaminated by the organisms that are natural to the rectum. Cystitis is painful. It is characterized by frequency, burning upon urination, and elevated temperature. Antibiotics, increased fluids, and rest are measures to treat cystitis. In females, the importance of avoiding contamination and of wiping from the front to the back after voiding and defecating must be emphasized.

8. *Vaginitis.* Atrophy of the female reproductive tract progresses slowly but steadily after menopause, and atrophic vaginitis causes considerable distress for some elderly females. Three problems plague the shrinking vagina: thinning of the epithelium, decrease in estrogen production, and lack of acidity of the vaginal secretions. Left untreated, adhesions, infection, and dyspareunia can result.

9. *Cancer.* Cancer is the second major disorder of the aged. The genitourinary sites in women are:

vulva—leukoplakia (thickened white patches) often is the first sign; precancerous lesion

vagina—seldom a primary site; usually is involved secondarily

cervix—more common in women of menopausal age than in elderly women

uterus—endometrial cancer is common; endometrial polyps can be precancerous

ovaries—high incidence in aged women

bladder—seen in elderly women but more common in aged men

breast—a significant cause of cancer deaths in elderly women

Prophylaxis is emphasized: the Papanicolaou (Pap) smear, physical examination of the pelvic organs, and prompt investigation of any bleeding from the body's orifices are means of identifying and controlling cancer. The nurse can also encourage the elderly woman to learn how to do a breast self-examination and to do it monthly.

Genitourinary cancer sites in men are:

bladder—common cancer in the elderly, but significantly higher incidence in males; painless bleeding usually the first sign; linked to smoking

prostate—benign prostatic hypertrophy affects virtually all elderly males. The prostate can be examined by a physician during an annual checkup. Since urinary difficulty occurs mainly in men over 60, a physician's examination is necessary to determine whether the problem is benign prostatic hypertrophy or cancer of the prostate.

Nursing Measures and Procedures

Genitourinary problems are distressing, embarrassing, and annoying. Unfortunately they are often regarded philosophically and are accepted as "to be expected" because of advancing years. The danger is that what some people are passing off as caused by old age may be early warning signs of infection or malignancy.

Nurses need to take time to understand the geriatric patient. Many females over 65 had their babies at home and are fearful and suspicious in the unfamiliar hospital setting. Explaining procedures before they are done and respecting the patient's privacy go a long way in gaining cooperation.

Elderly men have difficulty in accepting significant symptoms and they may misinterpret medical advice. Any threat to masculinity is intolerable—at any age. The nurse's attitude can generate trust and motivation. Shame and fear make patients delay the investigation of symptoms. Education of the genitourinary patient, particularly by stressing the seven danger signs of cancer, can help prevent the tragic outcome of neglect that so often shows up in physicians' offices and in hospitals.

Assisting with the Pelvic Examination

Nurses can gain their patients' confidence and cooperation by giving simple explanations of what is to be done and why. When assisting the physician at the pelvic examination of an elderly patient, be sure that the proper equipment is at hand, that there is adequate lighting, and that privacy is assured.

Purposes
to prepare the patient for a pelvic examination
to take care of any specimens obtained

Equipment

bath blanket	sterile glove	materials that may
speculum	small hand towel	be needed for tak-
lubricant	small pillow	ing specimens

Sequence
1. identify patient; introduce self; explain procedure; have patient void; cleanse perineal area
2. position patient on examining table, legs in stirrups, pillow under head
3. drape with bath blanket after patient has hips brought down to end of table
4. reassure patient; adjust lights for physician
5. if Papanicolaou smear is to be taken, have swabs, glass slide, and fixative ready for physician
6. be sure specimen is properly labeled
7. dry perineal area with hand towel (there may be some traces of lubricant left from the speculum)
8. remove both legs simultaneously from stirrups
9. encourage elderly patient to sit for a few minutes before getting off examining table
10. help patient with putting on gown or assist with dressing if needed

Giving the Bedpan and Urinal
Bedpans, urinals, and commodes are used to provide for a patient's elimination and to aid in measuring output. Patients should be given the opportunity to use a bedpan or urinal before starting any treatments and before leaving the room for trips to

x-ray and physical therapy. The nurse should also offer the bedpan before each meal, when the patient awakens in the morning, and at bedtime.

Purposes
to give and remove a bedpan and urinal
to measure and record output
to collect a specimen

Equipment

bedpan or urinal	soap	toilet tissue
cover	towel	basin of water
		room deodorizer

Sequence

1. identify patient; introduce self; screen patient; elevate bed to level of comfort
2. run hot water over rim of pan if necessary to warm it
3. if patient is able, have him help by digging his heels into the bed and pushing up on his elbows while the nurse places a hand under his lower back and slides bedpan or urinal into place
4. for a helpless patient, roll patient on to side with the aid of another person; position pan against buttocks and roll patient back on pan; *then* elevate bed after patient is positioned correctly
5. leave patient with call signal and toilet tissue at hand
6. remove bedpan as it was given, remembering to use bedpan cover
7. roll helpless patient on side, wrap tissue around hand and wipe from pubic area to anus; use wet cloth if necessary; inspect the perineum carefully to check for redness or excoriation
8. do not discard contents of any bedpan until you are sure contents   don't have to be measured *or* that a specimen doesn't have to be taken
9. collect specimens as per hospital policy, being careful not to let toilet tissue get into bedpan
10. offer basin of water, soap, towel to patient or wash his hands if he is unable to do so.

11. clean and replace equipment and wash *your* hands

ADDITIONAL INFORMATION: A way to clean an incontinent patient is to have the patient sit on the bedpan and pour a quantity of warm water over the perineal area. This helps prevent skin problems and contributes to a feeling of cleanliness.

Very thin patients should have the bedpan padded with a folded towel as a comfort measure. When there is a problem in sitting on a bedpan either because of dressings, contractures, or casts, a fracture pan should be offered.

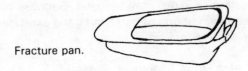

Fracture pan.

The nurse should remember that it can be very embarrassing or people to have to use a bedpan. And, while it would be ideal or male patients to be given bedpans and urinals by orderlies, it sn't always possible. A cheerful, matter-of-fact attitude demonstrates a sincere interest in the patient's well-being and essens self-consciousness.

Bladder Training

Urinary incontinence is as distressing to patients as it is to nurses. The first step in a program of bladder training is to have the patient evaluated by a physician. Is the incontinence caused by a urinary tract infection or by some disorder or disease? Is there some mechanical problem as in the case of calculi or an enlarged prostate? Often the question is one of communication. Can the patient tell the nurse he has to void? Aphasics can't. The most frustrating situation probably occurs when the patient knows he has to void but the siderails are up and his light isn't answered on time—so he wets the bed. Once the cause of incontinence is established, certain general rules for bladder training may be followed.

1. see that the patient has an adequate fluid intake (2500 ml daily)

2. record voidings to try to identify a pattern; involve the patient in the record keeping if this is possible

3. offer a bedpan or urinal periodically, especially first thing in the morning and after meals
4. keep bedding dry and keep patient's skin clean by washing with soap and water when incontinence has occurred
5. answer call lights promptly
6. apply ordered ointments to any perineal rashes
7. encourage the patient and praise successes

If the diagnosis is stress incontinence (escape of urine when coughing, laughing, or sneezing), the Kegel exercises, where the patient is taught to consciously contract and expand or relax the perineal muscles used in voiding, may be used. Success comes slowly and only after a long period of performing the exercises 50 times a day in series of five at a time.

Obtaining a Clean Catch Urine Specimen

At one time all specimens for a urine culture were obtained by catheterization. Within the last few years, however, clean catch specimens have been found acceptable for this laboratory test. The nurse should first determine whether "midstream" and "clean catch" are used synonymously. Then she should find out if the container must be sterile (many agencies use clean containers). Once there is a clear understanding of terms, the nurse may proceed to collect the specimen.

Equipment

sterile disposable "clean catch" pack

OR sterile collection container

antiseptic swabs
clean gloves
sterile bedpan or urinal (optional)

Sequence
1. identify patient; introduce self; explain procedure; screen patient
2. inspect perineal area to be sure external meatus is clean
3. wearing clean gloves, wash off external meatus area with antiseptic swabs (keep labia of female patient separated)
4. place female patient on bedpan and have her void a small amount into the pan; now, holding the sterile container at

the meatus, let the urine fall directly into it (*NOTE*: some agencies have patient void into a *sterile* bedpan and then collect the specimen; check policy of health care facility)
5. offer urinal to male patient; instruct him to void a small amount into urinal and then to void directly into the sterile specimen container
6. provide whatever aftercare is necessary
7. label specimen; record procedure; take or send specimen to laboratory

NOTE: There are many elderly patients who are capable of carrying out this procedure without the assistance of the nurse. Simply review the instructions to be sure the patient understands what is expected of him.

Recording Intake and Output

About two-thirds of the body's weight is water. It is important that the amount of fluid taken in by the body compensates for the amount of fluid used and excreted by the body. This is what fluid balance means.

The elderly adult needs about 2500 ml (about two- and a-half quarts) of oral fluids daily and the nurse should encourage adequate fluid intake. Some elderly people restrict their fluids for fear of incontinence or because they hope to avoid frequency and nocturia.

The body tolerates losing body weight better than losing body fluids. Fluids leave the body in urine, feces, respiration, perspiration, wound drainage, and vomitus.

A hospitalized patient may lose more fluid than is normal because of severe vomiting, diarrhea, and fever. An elderly patient will react to dehydration in the following ways: loss of skin turgor, dry mouth, elevated urea levels in the blood, and confusion. Inadequate fluids can also result in infections and constipation. Conversely, overhydration can pose a threat to the aged adult because of decreased renal and cardiovascular functioning with resulting collection of fluid in the tissues.

There are medical reasons for the physician to order the in-

take and output of the patient to be measured. It is helpful in mak
ing a diagnosis, in evaluating the condition of a patient, and i
monitoring the action of drugs.

Patients who are edematous may be on diuretics. Nursing
considerations here (besides recording of I & O) are daily weight
taking and replacement of lost electrolytes. Electrolytes are salt
in the blood—mainly potassium, sodium, calcium, and bicar
bonate. Diuretics are used to eliminate sodium, which is the
cause of fluid retention. To some extent, potassium is als
eliminated. Potassium may be replaced by medications or b
eating foods that are rich in potassium, namely, bananas, raisins
orange juice, cabbage, and celery.

Intake and output records must be accurate. For example, if
120 cc glass of juice is on the patient's tray and he drinks onl
half of it, 60 cc is recorded. Intake fluids recorded are:
 fluids administered parenterally
 water, juices, soft drinks, milk
 tea, coffee
 soups
 jello
 ice cream
 dietary supplemental drinks (Ensure, Sustecal, and so on)

Output recorded includes urine, feces, perspiration (sligh
moderate, profuse), any vomitus, wound drainage, suctio
drainage.

Most agencies have the intake and output sheet taped to th
patient's door or to his bedside stand. Entries must be prompt, a
curate, and neat.

Purposes
to find out how much fluid has been gained or lost from the
 body
to determine whether the patient is dehydrated
to learn the results of fluid restriction
to keep an accurate record of fluids taken and excreted

Equipment
fluid balance record on patient's chart
intake and output sheet   calibrated gradua

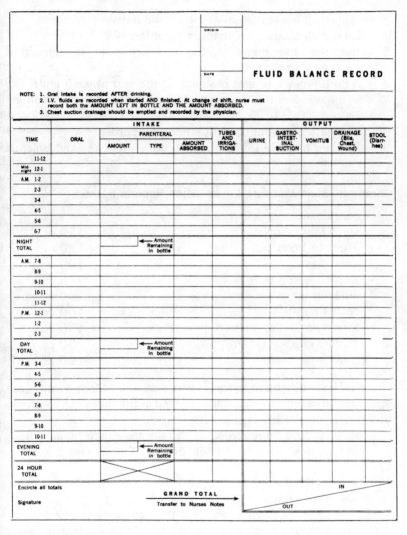

Fluid balance record.

Sequence
1. identify patient; explain procedure
2. encourage patient participation if feasible

3. record all liquids taken at meals and between meals
4. record all fluids administered parenterally
5. measure specimens voided into urinal or bedpan in a calibrated graduate
6. record Foley catheter drainage at the end of each shift
7. estimate wound drainage as scant, moderate, profuse; record
8. estimate perspiration if significant; record
9. be sure bedside I & O sheet is transferred to fluid balance record

Common Fluids Measured in cc when Recording Intake

container	cc
styro-foam cup	150 cc
4 ounce Dixie cup	120 cc
juice glass	100 cc
½ pint carton of milk	240 cc
drinking glass	200 cc
coffee cup	150 cc
serving of Jello, custard, junket	150 cc
1 Dixie cup ice cream	90 cc
small soup bowl	100 cc

NOTES: The above listing is just a sample. Most health care agencies have intake equivalents posted in the diet kitchen on the unit and/or on the I & O sheet itself.

Intake should be recorded each time the nurse takes a tray, glass, or pitcher away from the patient. Otherwise, it will be forgotten.

Foley Catheter Irrigation
There are physicians who feel that the best way to keep an indwelling catheter patent and draining is to force fluids. However, sometimes a Foley catheter irrigation is ordered.

An irrigation is a flush. Indwelling Foley catheters are irrigated to keep them patent and draining. At one time these irrigations were done routinely. Now, however, a physician's order is needed for a Foley irrigation. Strict sterile aseptic technique is used because irrigations can introduce pathogenic bacteria into the bladder. Since the sterile disposable equipment used for this procedure can be used only *one* time, it is more economical to use a sterile bulb or Asepto syringe and a sterile basin from the central supply room. Clean the equipment after you use it and return it to CSR.

When a catheter is disconnected from drainage tubing, the tubing is protected with a sterile catheter plug or a dry sterile dressing. Solution instilled is allowed to return by gravity. If clots obstruct drainage, the tubing may be milked *away* from the bladder.

It is essential for nurses to wash their hands before and after giving a bladder irrigation. Handwashing by patients is to be encouraged and provided for.

Purposes
to maintain a patent Foley catheter for urinary drainage
to promote patient comfort

Equipment

sterile disposable irrigation kit	sterile catheter plug
OR bulb or Asepto syringe and sterile basin	OR dry sterile dressing
	emesis basin (clean)
protective underpad	sterile irrigating solution
Alcowipe	

Sequence
1. identify patient; introduce self; explain procedure; screen patient
2. pour sterile irrigating solution into sterile basin
3. fold covers back far enough to just expose the catheter connected to the drainage tubing
4. place protective underpad under patient's hips; place emesis basin on bed
5. disconnect catheter; plug or cover tubing
6. fill syringe with prescribed amount of solution
7. instill solution slowly into catheter
8. permit solution to drain into emesis basin by way of gravity

9. repeat as ordered
10. wipe catheter end with alcohol and reconnect to drainage tubing
11. record the kind of solution and the amount used; describe the returns and how the patient tolerated the procedure.

NOTE: Many elderly patients have been told that this is a painful procedure. While it is true that in some surgical cases a bladder irrigation may produce bladder spasms, the patient should be reassured that every precaution will be taken to relieve distress and maintain comfort.

Urinary Meatus Care of Patient with Indwelling Foley Catheter

Urinary meatus care is given during the patient's bath. After the perineal area of the male or female patient has been thoroughly cleansed, proceed in the following way:
1. female patient—with labia well separated, apply antiseptic swab or bacteriocidal ointment to urinary meatus and around the indwelling Foley catheter
2. circumcised male—apply antiseptic swabs or bacteriocidal ointment to urinary meatus around Foley catheter
3. uncircumcised male—retract foreskin, apply swabs or ointment as above, then draw foreskin back over penis

Measures to Induce Voiding

The nurse should be familiar with many separate ways of helping the patient who has difficulty voiding. Inability to pass urine is uncomfortable and anxiety producing. The nurse's "bag of tricks" should include the following:
1. offer fluids, particularly warm drinks
2. have the patient blow bubbles through a straw in a glass of water (blowing relaxes the urethra)
3. let the patient listen to running water
4. place patient's hands in a basin of water
5. give patient a sitz bath (with physician's or supervisor's permission)
6. try to place the female patient in a sitting position—this position is the preferred position for females
7. if the male patient's condition permits, have him stand at the bedside

8. give a *warm* bedpan
9. place the patient on a bedpan and pour warm water over the genitalia
10. apply gentle downward pressure on the lower abdomen
11. have patient bend forward and rock gently
12. put spirits of peppermint *on* a cotton ball *in* a paper medicine cup *in* the bedpan (why this works is unclear—it may be that the vapors from the spirits of peppermint are warm and that this relaxes the sphincter muscle)

The most important move of all when trying to induce voiding is to help the patient relax. Providing privacy and encouragement help, as does a lessening of emotional tension. Frequently, all that is needed is to leave the patient *alone* for a few moments.

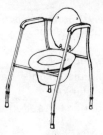

The bedside commode encourages bowel and bladder functioning.

Catheterization

Catheterization is the act of inserting a catheter (tube) into the urinary bladder to empty it of urine. The procedure is done for many reasons. For example, when surgery is to be done, an indwelling catheter may be ordered preoperatively to keep the bladder reduced in size. This allows the surgeon more room and/or allows for hourly urine measurement. Postoperatively, catheterization may be ordered when the patient is unable to void and all other measures to induce voiding fail. The procedure is also used to measure residual urine and to obtain specimens for some laboratory examinations. Frequently, indwelling catheters are placed in incontinent patients to keep them dry.

A Foley indwelling catheter has a separate valve that allows for the inflation of a 5 cc, 10 cc, or 30 cc balloon on the end of the catheter. When inflated, the balloon acts as an anchor to hold the catheter in the bladder. This catheter comes in sizes 14, 16, 18, 20, and 22.

A French catheter is a plain tube with no balloon and comes in sizes 10Fr., 12Fr., 14Fr., 16Fr., and 18Fr.

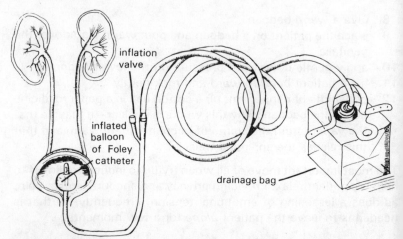

Kidneys, ureters, bladder, and inflated Foley catheter with drainage tube and drainage bag.

Equipment

sterile disposable catheterization kit
bath blanket
container for soiled equipment

goose neck lamp
extra pillows
tape

Sequence

1. identify patient; introduce self; explain procedure; screen patient
2. clean patient as necessary before beginning procedure if patient is incontinent
3. place patient in dorsal recumbent position and drape appropriately with bath blanket; pillows may be used under legs as a comfort measure
4. adjust light until perineal area is clearly seen
5. place protective underpad under hips, plastic side down
6. open catheterization kit near the work area, being sure to maintain a sterile field
7. put on sterile gloves
8. place drape from the kit on patient (sterile towels may be substituted)
9. lubricate tip of catheter liberally and keep catheter on sterile field

10. open container of cleansing solution and pour solution over all rayon balls in the kit *but one*
11. use *dry* rayon ball to protect fingers and separate labia; cleanse area using forceps to hold the moistened rayon balls (warn patient, "it's cold and wet")
12. discard all rayon balls and forceps in appropriate container—*not* on sterile field
13. tell patient to beathe deeply while you inset the catheter two to three inches for female patient and six to eight inches for male patient
14. hold catheter while urine is draining into container or into drainage bag (obtain specimen at this time if ordered)
15. allow no more than 500 cc to empty out of the bladder; if there is more urine in the bladder, simply clamp off the catheter and observe the patient for 20 minutes before proceeding with emptying the bladder
16. when urine stops flowing, pinch the catheter and withdraw it slowly if French catheter is used
17. if Foley catheter is used, reinflate the balloon using a pre-filled syringe
18. tape drainage tubing to leg, being careful not to kink tubing
19. leave patient clean, dry, and comfortable
20. record time of procedure, observations of urine, how patient tolerated procedure

NOTE: If a male patient is to be catheterized, Steps 1 to 10, *omitting* 3, are the same. The foreskin of an uncircumcised male is drawn back as the penis is cleansed. The penis is then raised nearly perpendicular to the body and the catheter inserted. The foreskin is then reduced and the procedure as outlined above is followed.

ADDITIONAL INFORMATION: Never catheterize a patient without an assistant or observer. Always be sure the lighting is adequate. The nurse must prepare to adapt all procedures to the individual patient. Catherterization is one of the more complicated procedures and demands practice and review in order to maintain sterile aseptic technique.

Vaginal Irrigation (Douche)

A douche is irrigation of the vagina; that is, an amount of fluid is instilled into the vagina and allowed to drain out via gravity. Physicians order douches preoperatively when certain types of surgery are scheduled. Sometimes douches are used to instill medication or to promote cleanliness when there is an abnormal discharge. A deodorizing douche may be ordered for a patient with a vesicovaginal fistula (abnormal passageway from the bladder to the vagina).

Routine home douching is discouraged as this can alter the natural flora of the vagina and cause dryness, irritation, and bacterial growth that may contribute to infection.

Equipment

warm irrigating solution and
  irrigating container with
  curved irrigating nozzle
OR sterile disposable douche
  kit

bedpan
protective underpad
clean gloves
bath blanket

Sequence

1. identify patient; introduce self; explain procedure; screen patient
2. have patient get in dorsal recumbent position; drape patient with bath blanket
3. pour solution into container
4. place patient on bedpan with protective underpad under hips
5. put on gloves
6. allow some solution to wash over perineum slowly to cleanse vulva and to accustom patient to temperature of solution
7. gently introduce curved irrigating tip into vagina, rotate slowly to cleanse all folds of vagina while solution flows in; control flow so it is not running too fast
8. when container is empty, dry perineum but keep patient on protective underpad as some solution may remain in vagina for a while

9.   care for equipment as per agency policy
10.   chart time of procedure, amount of solution, observation of
      returns, and how patient tolerated procedure

    NOTES: Agency policies differ. While a douche isn't a
sterile procedure, there may be times where sterile technique is
required.
    Before giving a douche, always have the patient empty the
bladder.

REVIEW

A. Multiple Choice (Select the Best Answer)
    1. Kidneys filter:
        a. nephrons
        b. nitrogenous wastes
        c. glomeruli
        d. calculi
    2. The ureters are:
        a. 6''-8'' long in the male
        b. 2''-3'' long in the female
        c. 12'' long tubes extending from the pelvis of the kidney to
            the bladder
        d. filtering units
    3. Nocturia means:
        a. decline in the amount of nephrons
        b. painful urination
        c. having to urinate during the night
        d. conscious contracting of the perineal muscles
    4. Cystitis means:
        a. kinking of a ureter
        b. fluid in the thorax
        c. fluid collecting in the pericardial sac
        d. inflammation of the urinary bladder
    5. Escherichia coli is a natural organism in the:
        a. colon
        b. urinary tract
        c. renal pelvis
        d. glomerulus

B. Matching Test (Match Column 1 with Column 2)

Column 1

a. pessaries

b. Kegel

c. calculi

d. prostatic hypertrophy

e. pathogenic bacteria

Column 2

_____ 6. often develop in immobilized patients

_____ 7. infect patients by way of indwelling catheters

_____ 8. worn in vagina to support uterus

_____ 9. exercise to eliminate stress in continence

_____ 10. nocturia is a symptom

C. Briefly Answer the Following Questions

1. What are some of the effects of inadequate fluid intake?
2. What are some of the reasons elderly people restrict their fluid intake?
3. What are some measures the nurse can take to help the patient void?
4. List five rules for bladder training of the incontinent patient.
5. Why do women have a much higher incidence of cystitis than men?

14

The Nervous System

Objectives

After completing this chapter, the student should be able to:

- describe the major purposes of the nervous system
- understand the changes that occur in the nervous system with aging
- assist the physician with neurologic examinations, spinal taps, and other examinations and procedures by preparing and caring for patients
- assess patients for neurological signs
- give general nursing care to patients with stroke, cerebrovascular disease, Parkinson's disease
- use the following words correctly

Vocabulary

The following words relate to the material in this chapter. Look up the ones you do not know or are not sure of.

adduction	ischemic	peripheral
aphasia	lethargic	postural hypotension
comatose	palpation	transient
foramen	percussion	vertigo

Anatomy Review

The brain and the spinal cord are the chief components of the nervous system, which is a vast communication network made up of nerve cells called neurons. The nervous system helps to regulate the functions and movements of the body.

All nerve tissue is extremely delicate. That is why the brain and the spinal cord are carefully protected by fluid, membranes, and bones.

Structures

Neurons. The neuron is an odd type of cell. Most of our cells reproduce; cells of the skin, bone, and blood are replaced when they wear out. But when neurons, the cells of the nervous system, die, they can't be replaced. A neuron is made up of a cell body and two types of extension—dendrites (one or more of them), which conduct nerve impulses to the neuron's cell body, and an axon which conducts nerve impulses away from the cell body. The axons are also referred to as nerve fibers.

Signals entering and leaving the body are passed via nerve fibers to the brain which, with its billions of neurons, analyzes the signals and transmits their meaning through other neurons, thereby giving direction to muscles.

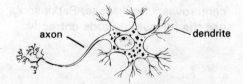

axon — dendrite

A nerve cell.

There are two types of nerves: *sensory nerves* that go from sense organs to the brain and *motor nerves* that go from the brain and spinal cord to the muscles. Some messages are conscious (voluntary) and some are involuntary. There are also reflex actions.

In a reflex action, the nerve impulses travel a special route called a reflex arc. For example, if you touch something hot, the impulse on the skin of your finger races along a sensory nerve to the spinal cord. There it generates another impulse that activates the muscle of your arm and you immediately pull your hand away. It's actually a shortcut whereby the muscles move before the brain knows why. Reflex actions protect the body from harm.

Special motor nerves make up the autonomic nervous system and they control the activities of our internal organs such as the heart, lungs, stomach, and intestines.

This is the way nerves carry messages. A stimulus, such as a pin, cotton ball, or ice cube, touches a nerve ending in the skin of the hand. This sets up an impulse (reaction) in the dendrite. The impulse speeds along the dendrite until it reaches the cell body. It then penetrates the cell body and exits through its axon away from the cell body to the dendrite of another neuron. Eventually it ends up in the brain. The brain interprets the impulse to be pain, a tickle, or perhaps a feeling of cold.

Spinal Cord. The spinal cord is a rope of nerve tissue about 16 inches long that is threaded through the protective bony arches of the vertebral foramina. It extends from the medulla through the vertebrae downward approximately four-fifths of the length of the spinal column.

Cranial Nerves. Twelve pairs of nerves branch off the brainstem and pass through the base of the skull into the brain. Thirty-one other pairs of nerves branch off the spinal cord at regular intervals between the vertebrae and reach all the organs of the body.

Nerves that reach upward from the spinal cord to the brain pass through the medulla oblongata (in the brainstem) where those from the left side of the body cross to the right side of the brain and vice versa. This is why the left side of the brain controls the right side of the body and the right side of the brain controls the left side of the body.

Structures of the Brain

The brain may be compared to a master computer which analyzes information and transmits orders to all parts of the body. It is made up of several components, each with its own functions:

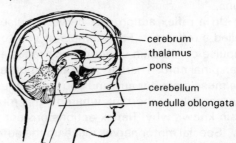

cerebrum
thalamus
pons
cerebellum
medulla oblongata

The brain.
Longitudinal section.

Cerebrum.   This is the largest part of the brain. It is composed of two hemispheres of convoluted (wrinkled) nerve tissue. The outer layer is called the cortex and is made up of "gray matter." The cerebrum helps with understanding, problem solving, memory, and thinking.

frontal lobe (thinking, memory, problem solving, understanding

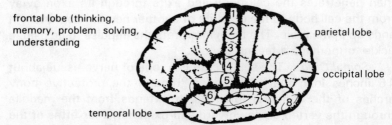

parietal lobe

occipital lobe

temporal lobe

Control zones of the cerebral cortex.

Nerve cells that control physical and mental activities are located in specific centers or zones of the cerebral cortex: (1) leg control; (2) body control; (3) arm control; (4) hand control; (5) face control; (6) speech; (7) hearing; (8) sight

Cerebellum.   The cerebellum is smaller than the cerebrum. It also is made up of two hemispheres. It is located at the back of the head. It coordinates our muscular activity.

Brainstem.   The brainstem connects the cerebrum with the spinal cord. Within the brainstem are: diencephalon, midbrain, pons, and medulla oblongata.

Diencephalon. This part of the brainstem contains the thalamus and the hypothalamus.

Midbrain. This is a short part of the brainstem just below the thalamus and above the pons. It sends signals on to the cerebrum along with the pons.

Pons. The pons passes signals from the cerebrum to the cerebellum.

Medulla Oblongata. This is the lower portion of the brainstem. It is a bulbous enlargement of the spinal cord that accepts and transmits nerve impulses which control breathing, digestive processes, and the circulation of the blood.

Four important concepts you should learn about this complex system of the body are:

1. All conscious activities (seeing, hearing, thinking, and so on) are controlled by the cerebrum.
2. Involuntary muscles such as those of the heart are controlled by the medulla oblongata.
3. Voluntary muscles are controlled by the cerebellum, although this control is automatic.
4. The spinal cord is the place where the nerve branches that reach out to all the organs of the body originate.

Age-Related Changes in the Nervous System

1. *Neuronal Loss.* There is a slow, gradual loss of neurons as people age. Neurons are lost by the thousands starting at age 25, but the picture isn't as depressing as it sounds because most of us function rather well despite the loss.
2. *Atherosclerosis.* In this country, almost everyone has some degree of atherosclerosis. This is probably due to a combination of genetic and environmental factors. A 75-year-old has blood flow to the brain that is about 80 percent of that of a 30-year-old. In advanced stages of atherosclerosis, however, plaque (a deposit of fatty material on the lining of the blood vessels) narrows the lumen of vessels and gradually occludes them. This serious impairment of blood flow to the brain can result in dizziness and stroke.

3.   *Behavioral Changes.*   Neuronal loss and atherosclerosis contribute to such behavioral changes as difficulty in remembering recent events, slowing of reaction responses, and difficulty in mastering motor skills. Old people who have trouble getting about or who are worried about what seems to be increasing helplessness are likely to be irritable. These reactions must be handled calmly, quietly, and constructively by the nurse. If an elderly person isn't rushed, or isn't confused by being moved into a new environment or by being subjected to a new routine, he usually can adapt to inevitable changes. Nurses must realize that most elderly persons *are* a bit slower mentally and physically than when they were younger. It may take longer for them to understand what is said and to accomplish a given direction. The key is to try to avoid pressure situations.

4.   *Cerebrovascular Disease.*   There are several types of cerebrovascular disease. The main types are cerebral infarction, transient ischemic attacks, intracranial hemorrhage and hypertension.

   Cerebral infarction, also called stroke, shock, or CVA, means that there is vascular disease that involves either a vein or an artery. The problem is caused either by a hemorrhage from a torn vessel or by an obstruction of the lumen of the vessel.

   Cerebral thrombosis is the usual cause of CVAs in the elderly. There is usually a previous history of arteriosclerosis. Some early warning signs may be vertigo, headache, lightheadedness, sudden falls without loss of consciousness ("drop attacks"), blurred vision, memory loss, and behavioral changes.

   Transient ischemic attacks (TIAs) are temporary dysfunctions of the central nervous system. Atherosclerotic vessels impair the circulation of the blood to a part of the brain and the patient experiences vertigo, loss of vision in one eye, aphasia, or confusion. The entire episode may last a few minutes or several hours. Treatment is either anticoagulant therapy (see Chapter 12) or reconstructive surgery of the blood vessel (endarterectomy). The person who has transient ischemic attacks has an increased chance of having a cerebral vascular accident. It's worth mentioning that cigarette smoking has a vasoconstrictive action and that the action of certain drugs, namely, antihypertensives and diuretics, can also cause poor cerebral circulation.

People with hypertension and arteriosclerosis are candidates for *intracranial or intracerebral hemorrhage.* The pressure builds up in the defective artery and the artery eventually ruptures and bleeds into the surrounding tissues. A clot forms and causes pressure on the site of the brain where the hemorrhage took place. Sometimes there are early warning signals, but often the attack is sudden. Symptoms vary widely, from severe headache, vertigo, and loss of consciousness to mental confusion, aphasia, nausea, and a feeling of weakness.

The initial effect of cerebral vascular accident is paralysis of one or both sides of the body. A right-sided paralysis (hemiplegia) indicates that the left side of the brain is involved. Occasionally the hemorrhage is slight, nerve damage temporary, and the paralysis not too serious.

Stroke patients have a characteristic appearance. Speech is indistinct, there's no muscle control on the affected side, and there may be no bowel or bladder control. These men and women suffer some mental confusion and are emotionally labile, i.e., they may laugh and cry inappropriately.

5. *Hypertension,* which is accompanied by inelasticity of blood vessels, is a significant cause of CVAs in the elderly. Any sign of epistaxis, disorientation, confusion, or poor memory should be investigated. A fine balance between blood pressure that is high enough to allow good circulation without being so low as to cause complications must be reached. Rest, sodium restriction, weight reduction (if indicated), and drug therapy can improve the condition of the hypertensive geriatric patient by helping to lower the blood pressure.

6. *Tumors.*   Most brain tumors occur in younger adults. Unfortunately, the few brain tumors that do occur in the aged

adult are often not diagnosed for a long time because the symptoms are so easily attributed to the aging process. Forgetfulness, personality changes, headaches, visual disturbances, and poor coordination are what we've grown to expect from the elderly. Most of the time the symptoms are attributed to arteriosclerosis; on other occasions ''senility'' is blamed.

Metastatic disease is prevalent in the elderly. A test that is done frequently on elderly patients is a brain scan. It is a painless procedure involving an intravenous injection of a substance that is picked up by lesions. These lesions are recorded by a scanner. What frightens patients is that they must remain perfectly still when this is being done and usually the head is immobilized. The scanner passes over the patient's head and seems very threatening. If the patient is prepared for this and reassured, the experience isn't anxiety provoking.

7. *Accident Proneness.* Progressive changes in vision and hearing, plus advancing neuromuscular changes make the elderly vulnerable to accidents. Falls are extremely common at home and in health care facilities. Postural hypotension, medication the patient is taking, momentary confusion, and furniture that is not in its usual place are a few of the causes of these falls. Simple preventive measures are needed. The environment at home and in the hospital must be made as hazard-free as possible. Routine safety precautions include:

> adequate lighting
> no scatter rugs or slippery floor surfaces
> bedrails at night
> clearly labeled medications
> handrails in bathtubs and on stairways
> electrical equipment in good working order (no frayed or
>   worn cords)

A younger person recovers quickly from injuries incurred by a fall. An elderly person is not only likely to have more serious consequences, but also to take a longer time convalescing.

8. *Tremor.* Tremor is occasionally observed in the elderly. A

fine trembling of the jaw or of the hand that increases when the person is hurried or under stress is sometimes referred to as "senile tremor." It is distinguished from the tremor of Parkinson's disease in that it is more rapid and is not medically significant.

9. *Parkinson's disease,* or paralysis agitans, is a degenerative disease of the nervous system. It involves a slow destruction of nerve cells. The symptoms are muscle weakness, tremor of the head and hands, shuffling gait, mask-like facial expression, and slow wooden speech.

Nursing Measures

Assisting with the Neurological Examination

A patient who is suspected of having a disease of the nervous system will be examined by a neurologist, that is, a physician who specializes in the field. A complete neurological examination may be done at intervals since it can be exhausting for the patient. After testing reflexes, gait, and special senses, the examiner will then order one or more of the diagnostic tests that are required to determine the cause of dysfunction. For example, if a spinal cord tumor is suspected, a myelogram may be ordered. These highly specialized diagnostic examinations will be discussed separately.

The nurse's responsibility with assisting at the neurological examination is to have the necessary equipment and materials ready for the physician and to prepare and reassure the patient. The patient should be clean, should have had an opportunity to void, and should have been given an explanation about the examination in keeping with his state of alertness at the moment.

Equipment

percussion hammer	colored yarn	applicators
straight pin	flashlight	something with a
safety pin	pocket watch	strong, nonirritat-
cotton ball or soft	something with a	ing smell (onion,
fine brush	definite but non-	tobacco, oil of
tuning forks	irritating taste	peppermint)
	(sugar, salt)	

Sequence for Testing Cranial Nerve Functions

1. olfactory: one nostril is closed; substance with a characteristic odor is held beneath the other nostril to test sense of smell; repeated with first nostril

2. optic: patient wears glasses if customary; color sense is tested with yarn; cover one eye and test for visual field by moving finger from behind head toward line of vision and note when patient first sees the finger; repeat

3.,4., and 6. oculomotor, trochlear, and abducent:
   a. patient is in semidarkened room; light is shone into eyes one at a time to see reaction
   b. patient holds head still and follows moving finger of examiner

5. trigeminal: test done with cotton and/or pinprick to check superficial sensations of face; heat and cold reaction also tested; corneal reflex tested with cotton strand (blinking)

7. facial: examiner places salty and sweet substances on tongue, asks for patient's reaction

8. acoustic: examiner tests hearing using pocket watch and various tuning forks

9.,10. glossopharyngeal and vagus: examiner tests for gag reflex with applicators

11. spinal accessory: patient rotates head, shrugs shoulders

12. hypoglossal: testing of movements of tongue

Other Tests

In addition to testing the cranial nerves, a neurological examination includes testing for:

Speech. The physician will ask the patient to identify ordinary objects (key, dollar bill, etc.), to follow simple commands ("raise your right hand"), and perhaps even read.

Muscle Status. Muscles are measured to check for symmetry of contraction. The use of palpation and a percussion hammer help to demonstrate muscle tone.

Gait. Gait observation involves having the patient walk forward, backward, and then walk with eyes closed.

Coordination. To test coordination, the physician may have the patient pour a glass of water from a pitcher, or have him close his eyes and try to touch his nose with a finger.

Reflexes. An example of reflex testing is the classic patellar reflex test in which the patellar tendon is hit with a percussion hammer. Another reflex is the plantar reflex, which is tested by stroking the sole of the foot to see if the toes flex or extend.

Sensitivity. This may be determined by pinching, squeezing, or pricking the patient to observe for reactions to pain. It can also include having the patient close his eyes and then tell the doctor which finger or toe is being held by the doctor. A strand of cotton may be used to touch the skin lightly to see if the patient can feel it.

Neurological Assessment

When working with patients who have a disease of the brain or spinal cord, you may be required to take "neuro signs." This means that the physician will order observations of neurological signs on a periodic basis.

Neurological signs include: orientation, bodily movements, pupillary reaction, speech, vital signs, affect.

Orientation. Does the patient know who he is? Where he is? What day it is?

Bodily Movements. Is the patient lethargic? Stuporous? Comatose? Does he voluntarily move his arms and legs? Is his muscle tone strong? Weak? Is his grip strong?

Pupillary Reaction. Do the patient's pupils constrict when a light is shone into the eyes? How long do they take to constrict? How much do they constrict? (Beam light on closed eye and then watch constriction of pupil when eye is opened; repeat for the other eye and compare pupillary reaction of second eye with first).

Speech. Can the patient speak? Is his speech clear? Is he confused? Aphasic? Can he identify ordinary objects or follow simple directions?

Vital signs. What are the patient's temperature, pulse, respirations, and blood pressure?

Affect. Does the patient appear depressed? Hostile? Tense or anxious? Or does he appear normal with appropriate comments and responses?

														NEUROLOGICAL ASSESSMENT SHEET
DATE ➤														
TIME ➤	AM PM	AM PM	AM PM	AM PM	AM PM	AM PM	AM PM	AM PM	AM PM	AM PM	AM PM	AM PM	AM PM	
L.O.C.														
ORIENTATION NAME														
PLACE														
DAY														
MOVEMENTS GRIP														
Ⓛ ARM														
R ARM														
Ⓛ LEG														
R LEG														
PUPIL SIZE R														
Ⓛ														
SPEECH CLEAR														
RUMBLING														
INCOHERENT														
APHASIC														
VITALS B.P.														
PULSE														
RESP.														
TEMP.														
MISC.														
NURSE'S SIGNATURE														

ABBREVIATIONS	ORIENTATION	MISCELLANEOUS ABBREVIATIONS	PUPIL CHART	
Q – QUIET	MOVEMENTS	= EQUAL	2 • 5 ● 8 ●	RB – REACT BRISKLY
D – DROWSY	I EXCELLENT	> STRONGER	3 • 6 ●	R – REACT
A – ALERT	II GOOD	< WEAKER		RS – REACT SLOWLY
C – CONFUSED	III AVERAGE		4 ● 7 ●	F – FIXED
SS – SLIGHTLY SLURRED	IV BELOW AVERAGE			

Neurological assessment sheet.

Other Examinations

There are other examinations you should become familiar with when caring for a patient with a disease of the nervous system. These include laboratory examination reports of the spinal fluid, x-ray studies, and computerized axial tomography (CAT scans).

Patients with neurologic disease are usually in pain, and almost always tense and anxious. The nurse's responsibility is to give physical care and also to lend emotional support through interest and concern. Eye contact, a caring attitude and simple answers to the questions that can be answered help to establish trust and confidence.

Cerebrospinal fluid is obtained for laboratory examinations by means of a lumbar puncture or a cisternal puncture. The lumbar puncture, or spinal tap, is more commonly used.

While health agency policies vary, and the nurse must familiarize herself with those of her particular agency, there are general steps she will take:

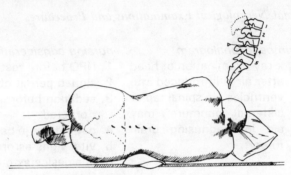

Position for lumbar puncture.

Lumbar Puncture (site: between L4 and L5 or L5 and S1)
1. obtain a signed permit from the patient for the procedure
2. prepare the puncture area (either shave or scrub as per physician's order)
3. position patient on his side, near edge of bed or examining table
4. assist patient to *hold* this position during lumbar puncture
5. give aftercare of patient as ordered (flat in bed, analgesics as ordered)
6. label specimen accurately and have it delivered to laboratory immediately

Cisternal Puncture (site: cisterna magna at base of brain)
This procedure is done if the physician is unable to do a spinal tap.

The basic steps are the same as for lumbar puncture except that the area prepped is the back of the neck.

Normal Characteristics of Cerebrospinal Fluid

appearance	clear
glucose	45-75 mg per 100 ml
total protein	15-45 mg per 100 ml
white cell count	0-5 lympocytes
	0 neutrophils

Special Neurological Examinations and Procedures

pneumoencephalogram

x-ray examination of head after air is introduced into ventricles via spinal tap or cisternal puncture; may aid in diagnosing brain tumor

nursing considerations
1. NPO before test
2. signed permit obtained
3. sedation before test as ordered
4. patient flat in bed after x-ray
5. vital signs as ordered
6. analgesics as ordered
7. icecap to head

arteriogram

x-ray examination of head after dye is injected into carotid artery; used to detect obstructions, aneurysms

1. signed permit obtained
2. sedation as ordered
3. vital signs
4. ice collar to injection site
5. neuro signs
6. watch for signs of shock (because of dye)

myelogram

injection of dye into spinal canal; used for diagnosing herniated disks, spinal cord tumors

1. NPO before test
2. signed permit obtained
3. back prepped
4. sedation as ordered
5. flat in bed after x-ray
6. vital signs
7. analgesics

brain scan
   an intravenous injection of radioisotope into brachial artery, used to detect brain lesions

nursing considerations
no special preparation before scan;
no special care after scan

electroencephalogram
   (EEG) observation of brain wave activity after attaching electrodes to head; helps locate blood clots, tumors, and indicates brain death

no preparation; after EEG shampoo to remove electrode jelly from hair

computerized axial tomography
   (CAT scan) patient lies on back, head inside scanning unit; many sections of brain studied in minute detail; no discomfort or risk; detects tumors, brain injuries, bone abnormalities

no preparation, no special care after scan

The Stroke Patient

The onset of a CVA is frequently sudden and it demands attention to the immediate needs of the patient, i.e., maintaining an open airway, protecting the patient from injury, recording vital signs, monitoring neurological signs, and administering IVs and medications.

The convalescent stage is usually prolonged and requires a sustained physical and emotional effort on the part of the nurse and the patient's family. The patient needs continual emotional support as well as frequent praise for the progress being made. Self-care should be encouraged as soon as the patient can tolerate the high Fowler's position and has arm movement and hand grasp.

Rehabilitation starts early. Nursing care is directed toward preventing deformities, regaining the use of the affected side, and leading the patient toward independence in the activities of daily living.

The three chief, and sometimes life-threatening, complications are: decubitus ulcers, pulmonary infection, and urinary tract infection. The immobilized patient needs meticulous skin care, frequent change of position, and proper body alignment. Oral hygiene and range of motion exercises must also be given. Pulmonary problems can be prevented by having the patient cough, deep breathe, and do breathing exercises, if possible, and by judicious oral and nasopharyngeal suctioning.

After the immediate nursing needs are met, efforts must be made to prevent flexion deformities by positioning and body alignment. Foot drop, external rotation of the hip, adduction of the affected shoulder, and contractures of the affected hand must be prevented through positioning and exercises.

The following are general measures you should be familiar with when planning the nursing care of the convalescent CVA patient.

1. prevent hypostatic pneumonia by changing the patient's position every two hours; encourage coughing and deep breathing if the patient is responsive
2. prevent contractures and other deformities by using hand rolls, trochanter rolls, ROM exercises, footboards, and so on
3. encourage good nutrition and hydration; note I & O
4. maintain good skin condition by keeping the bed linen clean and dry, changing the patient's position frequently, and giving back rubs with position changes
5. encourage the patient's participation in whatever ADL he is capable of even if it's in a very small way; example—let him handle a piece of toast while being fed breakfast
6. get the patient out of bed and out of his room as soon as this is permitted to expose him to the stimuli of other sights and sounds
7. allow the family to participate in the patient's care by feeding him, wheeling him in a wheelchair, caring for his hair, and so on
8. follow the plans of the physical therapist, speech therapist,

and occupational therapist to insure reinforcement of therapy

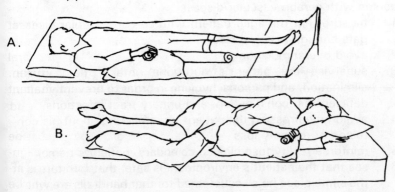

Positions for nonambulatory stroke patients in bed. A.—Pillow is placed next to body on paralyzed side. Hand roll is placed under hand on paralyzed side to keep fingers open; trochanter rolls are used to support the patient's leg on the paralyzed side so the leg won't rotate outwardly. B.—Pillow is used to support paralyzed arm. Another pillow supports the paralyzed leg.

There are over 200,000 CVA deaths a year—11 percent of all U.S. deaths. In addition, there are over two million Americans who have had one stroke and will have another.

Some basic warning signals of impending stroke are:
1. sudden weakness, numbness, or tingling in face or extremity
2. loss or slurring of speech
3. double vision or loss of vision, particularly in one eye
4. unexplained headaches
5. sudden dizziness or weakness
6. personality or behavioral changes

Medical attention should be sought if any of the above signs are experienced or observed.

Anyone can be a stroke victim, but some people are more vulnerable than others. Prevention includes: 1) control of existing hypertension; 2) seeking medical attention for any of the warning signs of stroke; 3) adhering to a nutritionally sound diet; 4) stopping smoking.

Nursing Measures for Patients with Cerebrovascular Disease

The following are some general measures for the care of the aged person with cerebrovascular disease:

1. be sure that the aged patient with cerebrovascular disease gets enough rest and sleep
2. avoid overstimulation
3. supervise the patient's nutritional intake, fluid intake, elimination, and personal hygiene in order to prevent vitamin deficiencies, constipation, and urinary tract infections
4. avoid embarrassing the patient by remarking about his confusion or memory loss
5. reinforce reality (use clocks, calendars, patient's name)
6. see that the patient's environment is safe; that furniture is in the same place he's accustomed to; that handrails are where needed; that he is suitably clothed when going out
7. pay attention to the patient as an individual; comment about the weather, the seasons, his appearance; this lets him know you care and also reinforces security

Nursing Measures for the Patient with Parkinson's Disease (Paralysis Agitans)

Patients with parkinsonism may not be seen by the medical/surgical nurse until they have endured the disease for years. When they are hospitalized, it is often due to a secondary infection; they may have increased stiffness and weakness. While there is no cure, medication, surgery, and physical therapy are the three methods of treatment. Effective nursing care focuses on controlling rigidity and preventing contractures.

Nursing Care

1. keep the skin scrupulously clean, using lotion on dry areas
2. encourage frequent oral hygiene where there is drooling
3. provide a nutritionally adequate diet; encourage fluids; assist with feeding if needed, but allow the patient to do as much for himself as possible; see that patterns of elimination are established
4. encourage active and passive exercise such as walking,

movement of arms, squeezing sponges or balls, and ROM for patients confined to bed

5. see that the patient gets enough rest and sleep; reduce stress

6. observe, report, and document changes in patient's condition; example—report any temperature elevation since this could be the beginning of an infection

7. encourage the family; be an interested listener to those who live with this long-term disability

REVIEW

A. Multiple Choice (Select the Right Answer)

1. The chief components of the nervous system are:
   a. neurons and dendrites
   b. axons and the brain
   c. spinal cord and neurons
   d. brain and spinal cord

2. Autonomic nerves control:
   a. sense organs
   b. internal organs
   c. peripheral nervous system
   d. central nervous system

3. The part of the brain which helps us to understand, solve problems and to remember is:
   a. cerebrum
   b. cerebellum
   c. medulla
   d. pons

4. As we age, we all have:
   a. behavioral changes
   b. neuronal loss
   c. tremor
   d. hypotension

5. An early warning sign of CVA is:
   a. irritability
   b. hyperpyrexia
   c. drop attack
   d. memory loss

B. Matching Test (Match Column 1 with Column 2)

Column 1	Column 2
a. hemiplegia	_____6. dizziness
b. vertigo	_____7. paralysis on one side of the body
c. hypostatic	_____8. high blood pressure
d. symmetry	_____9. lack of movement
e. hypertension	_____10. evenness

C. Briefly Answer the Following Questions

1. Name three ways of reinforcing reality.
2. List ways of encouraging active and passive exercises for the patient with Parkinson's disease.
3. When should ROM be omitted?
4. What are some basic warning signals of stroke?
5. What are some ways to reduce the likelihood of stroke?

15

The Endocrine System

Objectives

After completing this chapter the student should be able to
- better understand the endocrine system
- describe how diabetes mellitus occurs
- understand the roles of insulin and oral hypoglycemics in stabilizing diabetes mellitus
- recognize diabetic emergencies and know what to do should they occur
- give insulin and test urine for sugar and acetone
- teach diabetic patients how to care for themselves
- understand the comparative costs of the various diabetic medications
- use the following words correctly

Vocabulary

The following words relate to the material in this chapter. Look up the ones you do not know or are not sure of.

acetone   hyperglycemia   polydipsia

acidosis	hypoglycemia	polyphagia
benign	ketosis	polyuria
beta cells	kilogram	reagent
glucagon	metabolism	retinopathy
hormone	pathologic	syncope

Anatomy Review

A gland is a structure which produces and secretes certain chemical substances that are necessary for the functioning of the body's organs. There are two kinds of glands: exocrine and endocrine.

Exocrine glands have ducts (tiny tubes) through which their secretions pass directly to the area of the body that needs them. Some examples of exocrine glands are: lachrymal glands, salivary glands, mammary glands (in females only), intestinal glands, sebaceous glands, and bulbo urethral glands.

Endocrine glands, on the other hand, are ductless—their secretions are discharged directly into the blood or lymph. The major endocrine glands are:

 adrenals
 gonads (ovaries in the female and testes in the male)
 pancreas
 parathyroid
 pituitary
 thyroid

Two other endocrine glands are: 1) the *thymus,* which secretes one hormone that promotes cellular reproduction and growth and another that affects lymphatic tissue and immune mechanisms, and 2) the *pineal gland,* which secretes a hormone that acts or the hypothalamus and pituitary glands. In addition, there are other ductless glands whose functions are relatively minor or not clear.

The pancreas is both an exocrine and an endocrine gland. It channels pancreatic fluid into the digestive tract and its islets of Langerhans secrete the hormone insulin directly into the bloodstream.

Endocrine glands, together with the nervous system, govern the body's systems, but the endocrine glands also govern each other. The best example of this is the pituitary—the master gland

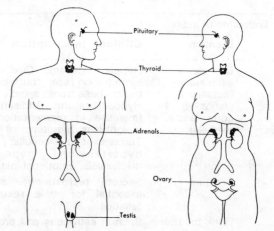

Location of the major endocrine glands. Courtesy of C.V. Mosby Co.

of the body. The pituitary hangs by a stem from the base of the diencephalon and fits into the sphenoid bone at the base of the skull just above the roof of the mouth. It secretes a variety of hormones, including those that influence: growth; sexual development; some gonad, thyroid, and adrenal functioning; milk production after childbirth; and some kidney functioning.

Age-Related Changes

There are not many disorders of aging that are directly caused by the malfunctioning of the adrenal glands, although as a person grows older he may fall victim to a malfunctioning gland just as a younger person may. However, with age there is a gradual decrease in thyroid, parathyroid, and adrenal hormone secretion. Changes in gonad secretions are discussed in the chapter on the urinary and reproductive systems.

There is, however, one hormone-related disease that is common among the aged, and that is diabetes mellitus, which will be discussed in this chapter. But, before discussing diabetes, it is important to review some common endocrine disorders which the nurse is likely to see in her work. The following table reviews typical malfunctions caused by over- or under-secretion of the glands.

The Major Endocrine Glands

Gland	Location	Clinical Information
Adrenals	One above each kidney (actually 2 glands—a. cortex and a. medulla)	Hypercorticalism: Cushing's syndrome (moon face; "buffalo" hump on back; obese trunk; spindly legs) Hypocorticalism: Addison's disease (increase in pigmentation of skin, weight loss, hypotension) Tumors of a. medulla: can cause hypertension, hypoglycemia, diaphoresis, emotional instability
Gonads: Testes in male	Scrotum	Secrete testosterone, a hormone essential for male sexual characteristics
Ovaries in female	Flank the uterus in pelvis	Secrete estrogens and progesterone, hormones that govern ovulation and female sexual development
Pancreas	Behind the stomach	Double duty gland: exocrine because it secretes digestive juice, and endocrine because it secretes the hormone insulin via islets of Langerhans; hyposecretion of the islets of Langerhans causes diabetes mellitus
Parathyroid	Attached to and behind the thyroid	Hyperparathyroidism: destruction of bone; pathologic fractures; kidney stones Hypoparathyroidism: patient feels tingling in extremities; muscle spasms; seizures; treat by regulating calcium and phosphorous
Pituitary	Base of brain	Hyperpituitarism: frequently caused by tumors; may result in acromegaly giantism, Cushing's disease Hypopituitarism: dwarfism; reproductive problems
Thyroid	In neck	Goiter: enlarged thyroid; may be due to lack of iodine in diet, inflammation or hyper- or hypofunction of thyroid Thyroiditis: inflammation of thyroid caused by bacteria or virus Tumors: usually benign in younger patients Hyperthyroidism: Graves' disease caused by overproduction of thyroid hormone; patient has exophthalmos, weight loss, enlarged thyroid, nervousness

Hypothyroidism: caused by lack of thyroid gland; in women over 60, myxedema is common, causing weight gain, dry skin and hair, sluggishness; cretinism in children with stunted growth, mental retardation

Diabetes Mellitus

Diabetes mellitus is a chronic disease that is characterized by a disturbance in the metabolism of carbohydrates, proteins, and fats.

There is a decrease in the use of glucose by cells and the blood sugar rises (hyperglycemia). When blood sugar reaches a certain high level, the kidneys excrete the excess and glucose appears in the urine (glycosuria).

The sugar in the urine upsets normal kidney function and causes more water and electrolytes to be excreted. Excessive urine output (polyuria) causes the person affected to become dehydrated and extremely thirsty (polydipsia).

One result of abnormal fat metabolism is an increase in ketones, the byproducts of fat metabolism. Excess ketones may be excreted in the urine (ketouria) but they can reach levels whereby they are not all safely excreted and this condition is called acidosis. A person with acidosis can deteriorate into diabetic coma and die.

Diabetes mellitus may be growth-onset (juvenile diabetes) or maturity-onset (beginning in adulthood). Since juvenile diabetics usually lack insulin, they need to take insulin because it decreases blood sugar levels. Maturity-onset diabetics have some insulin circulating in their blood and these people often respond well to oral hypoglycemic drugs and diet therapy.

Insulin (a protein) is a hormone secreted by the islets of Langerhans, which are the endocrine portion of the pancreas. In the islets of Langerhans there are two types of cells: alpha cells, which secrete glucagon, and beta cells, which secrete insulin.

Insulin causes a decrease in blood sugar levels because it apparently aids the movement of glucose through cell membranes, which causes the sugar molecules to leave the blood and go into the cells.

When blood glucose levels elevate, insulin is released. When blood glucose levels fall, insulin is not secreted.

Identifying Diabetes in the Elderly

It isn't easy to identify diabetes in the elderly. The standard symptoms that nurses have been taught to recognize (polydipsia, polyuria, and polyphagia) may not exist. Instead, there may be other physical problems that not only coexist with the diabetes but also demand more attention. Some examples are stroke, glaucoma, digestive disturbances, and infections.

The common urine test for sugar and acetone isn't a good indication of hyperglycemia in the aged, either. It's entirely possible for the patient to be hyperglycemic and yet not have it show up in urine tests. Glucose tolerance tests are the most accurate. Note the "s" in the word "tests." More than one is recommended to eliminate the chance that the results are false. Factors that confuse glucose tolerance test findings are: prolonged bed rest, malnutrition, severe illness, and certain drugs, for example, diuretics. It's clear that an accurate medical history is essential for diagnosis and treatment.

Complications of Diabetes

Complications are a serious risk to the elderly diabetic. Heart attacks and cerebral vascular accidents can occur as a result of untreated hypoglycemia. The usual symptoms of hypoglycemia (fatigue, weakness, anxiety, headache, vertigo, sudden hunger, irritability, and syncope) may not be apparent in the aged adult, and what the nurse might see instead are the stereotypical symptoms of "senility," e.g., confusion, disorientation, thick speech, inappropriate responses, and so on.

The older diabetic is very susceptible to infections. Nursing care should stress skin hygiene in general and foot care in particular. Skin injuries heal slowly and, if neglected, infections, gangrene, and even amputations are possible results.

Visual impairment (diabetic retinopathy) is a severe and progressive complication of the disease. The capillaries which supply the retina develop aneurysms. Thrombosis and/or hemorrhage follow. This bleeding into the vitreous humor can develop into fibrous bands that gradually shorten and pull on the retina, causing it to become detached. The patient needs support, encouragement, and instruction in maintaining independence as much as possible.

Nursing Responsibilities and Measures

Recognizing the Symptoms of Insulin Reaction and Acidosis

Nurses should be able to recognize the symptoms of insulin reaction (insulin shock) and acidosis (diabetic coma). They are both serious conditions and require prompt treatment.

Insulin Reaction (hypoglycemia)
(caused by too much insulin or too little food, or by stress, vomiting, diarrhea, unusual activity)

Symptoms:
hunger
diaphoresis
dizziness
pale, moist skin
blurred vision
nervousness
tremor
convulsion
coma

Treatment:
fruit juice with added sugar, hard candy, glucagon

Acidosis (hyperglycemia)
(caused by lack of insulin and accumulation of ketone bodies, or by stress, illness, or injury)

Symptoms:
nausea, vomiting
drowsiness
confusion
characteristic sweet, fruity odor to breath
rapid pulse
abdominal pain
restlessness
flushed face
coma

Treatment:
contact a physician, who will order blood and urine tests. When results are reported, a rapid acting insulin will be ordered.

NOTE: Never attempt to give anything orally if the patient is unable to swallow. Contact a physician.

Testing Urine for Sugar and Acetone

In order to determine the amount of insulin a patient requires, the nurse may be asked to test his urine for sugar and acetone. Frequently she is also asked to teach the patient how to do these tests. There are a number of tests available, all of them with easy-to-follow manufacturers' instructions, and all of them relatively easy to do. There are two basic types:

1.   A tablet is dropped into the urine specimen for a specified period of time after which the color of the urine is compared with a color chart.
2.   A strip of treated paper is held in a specimen of urine for a specified period of time and its color is then compared with a color chart.

Insulin

Insulin has been available commercially for over half a century. It is prepared from substances extracted from the pancreases of cattle and pigs and is manufactured as "U-40," with 40 units of insulin in one cc, and as "U-80," with 80 units of insulin in one cc. While the two concentrations are still on the market, they are being phased out and probably will disappear within five years. One reason is that patients sometimes switch from one insulin to another without consulting their physicians. This means that they can be injecting twice as much or half as much insulin as before! A simpler, less error-prone concentration is U-100. This means that there are 100 units of insulin in one cc. If the one cc insulin syringe is filled, it will contain 100 units. Since we measure liquids in cc's and in tenths of cc's, the feeling is that the development of U-100 syringes and insulin will decrease medication errors.

REMEMBER: A unit of insulin is a unit of insulin whether packaged as U-40, U-80, or U-100. This makes the change easy. The person who takes insulin needs only buy U-100 insulin of whatever kind, along with U-100 syringes from the several convenient types available. On the U-100 scale, the patient measures exactly the same number of units he has been taking.

How to Give Insulin

Insulin is injected subcutaneously at a 45° angle or at a 90° angle. The injection site is wiped with an alcohol sponge and the skin is stretched before inserting the needle. After insertion, aspirate to be sure the needle is not in a blood vessel. Inject the insulin. If the patient has little subcutaneous tissue, the skin should be pinched rather than stretched.

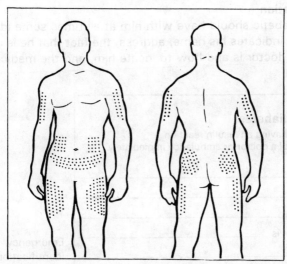

Sites for insulin injection. A different place should be chosen every day. It hurts less that way and is easier on the skin. One should never inject into a blood vessel that can be seen. Courtesy of Monoject.

Oral Hypoglycemics
There are now medications for lowering the blood sugar of diabetics that can be taken by mouth. They are called the oral hypoglycemics and do not contain insulin. Since, instead, they activate insulin release from the beta cells, they are effective in people who have some insulin reserve, including the adult onset individual who develops diabetes after the age of 40.

A second group of hypoglycemic agents, the biguanides, behave a little differently. These drugs affect glucose absorption and the production of glucose.

Only a physician decides whether the elderly diabetic needs insulin therapy or oral hypoglycemics. Some cases of diabetes can be controlled by oral hypoglycemics alone. However, these can be more expensive than insulin and that's a serious consideration for someone on a fixed income.

The Patients' Guidelines for Taking Oral Hypoglycemic Agents, shown on the opposite page, can be photocopied and given to patients.

Identification
Every diabetic should have with him at all times some identification that indicates his name, address, the fact that he is diabetic, who his doctor is and how to locate him, and the medication he takes.

I have diabetes!
I may be having an insulin reaction. Please call a doctor or ambulance immediately.
Name _____
Phone _____
Address _____
My doctor is _____
Phone _____
My hospital is _____
My medication is _____

Emergency identification card for diabetics. Courtesy of The Upjohn Company.

Teaching the Older Diabetic to Live with the Disease
Since diabetes mellitus is incurable, most patients feel angry on learning that they have the disease. They resent the fact that nature has singled them out for this disagreeable burden. They may be overwhelmed with feelings of anxiety. These are natural reactions to the fear of the unknown.

The nurse's responsibility for educating the diabetic patient is twofold: to teach him to understand his disease, and to be sure that he can competently care for himself.

Before planning any teaching, stop to consider that the patient probably has been getting along for 60 or more years doing things *his* way. Habits and lifestyles are hard to change and they won't be changed unless there's a motivation to change them. The nurse has to get to know her patient—his patterns of living, his educational background, and his limitations. Is the patient's hearing impaired? Is his vision satisfactory? Is there any evidence of arthritis in his fingers that would make it difficult to manage a syringe or uncap a bottle of tablets? Most important, how

---

Patients' Guidelines for Taking Oral Hypoglycemic Agents.

1. Remember to take your pills from one-half to one hour before meals unless your doctor directs otherwise. This will give the pills time to be absorbed in your system before food enters your bloodstream and raises the amount of glucose in the blood.

2. Get your doctor's approval before you switch from one pill to another. One tablet of one drug will not always give the same results as one tablet of another drug, even though they have the same amount of milligrams which are equal in strenght. Let your doctor determine the correct amount of milligrams for you. Each drug has a maximum amount that is considered effective. Taking more than this amount may increase the number of side effects.

3. Report all side effects to your doctor. Diarrhea, nausea, and loss of appetite may be due to the drug causing an irritation in the stomach. Skin rashes seem to occur most often with chlorpropamide (Diabinese).

4. Know the symptoms of hypoglycemia, low blood sugar caused from the stimulation of too much insulin: confusion, headache, hunger, nervousness, and pale, moist skin. Keep a concentrated source of sugar, such as a candy bar, on hand to curtail this reaction.

5. Beware of reactions with other drugs. Always check with your doctor or pharmacist before you combine a new medicine with your treatment for diabetes. If you drink alcohol while on these drugs, you may experience an unpleasant reaction such as flushing, nausea, and rapid heartbeat. The oral hypoglycemic agent prevents the alcohol from being broken down in the body.

6. Other drugs, such as steroids (Prednisone), estrogens, diuretics, Dilantin, Inderal, and the decongestants which are found in many cough and cold medictions, may interact with oral agents or interfere with diabetic control.

motivated is the patient? If he's too depressed to care, or too fearful to comprehend, these negative emotions must be relieved before any effective teaching can be done.

When explaining diabetes to a patient, it is best to have a family member present. After making the patient comfortable and removing distractions, present the information as simply as possible. At the outset, only the fundamental and most important facts should be mentioned. Detailed information about the pancreas and carbohydrate metabolism won't benefit the old person who has a poor memory and is hard of hearing. It would be better to concentrate on diet, medication, and urine testing.

There are vast quantities of printed explanations, instructions, and suggestions available for diabetic patients, but many of them have limitations — for example, they may be printed in small type, making it difficult for the visually impaired to read them, or they may be too technical for the patient to comprehend. The nurse has to make a special effort to adapt teaching aids to each patient.

The nurse should become familiar with the many useful aids for the visually impaired diabetic. There is, for example, MEGA-DIASTIX, a king-sized version of the Diastix test for urine glucose. It is designed to make it easier for visually impaired diabetics to do their own urine testing. The instructions are given in large type to make reading easier, and the reagent area of MEGA-DIASTIX is the same test material used for Diastix except that it is about three-fourths of an inch square. MEGA-DIASTIX is only available directly from the Ames Division of Miles Laboratories, Inc. Each kit contains 50 tests. The kit may be ordered from Ames Order Services Dept., P.O. Box 70, Elkhart, Indiana 46515. Ames also manufactures a scale magnifier that easily slips over an insulin syringe and makes accurate reading of dosages easier.

Good teaching includes reinforcement. When instructing an elderly person whose reaction time is slow and whose memory is poor, reinforcement is doubly important. The nursing care plan should indicate which important aspects of diabetic teaching need emphasis and how this is to be done by each member of the health care team.

Diabetic Nutrition

Since a patient's insulin needs are determined by exercise, emotion, diet, infection, and other factors, it is important to stabilize as many of these factors as possible. As a result, the diet should be controlled; indeed, diet is the basis of diabetic therapy. For more on diabetic nutrition, see Chapter 7, pages 110-113 .

Foot Care

Virtually all elderly diabetics have some degree of arteriosclerosis. The problems of peripheral vascular disease are intensified by this deterioration in circulation; the dependent extremities are especially vulnerable. This is why foot care is so important. Patients should be taught the following foot tips:

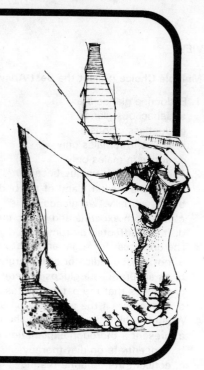

Foot Tips for the Diabetic

NEVER cut corns or calluses with a razor blade or knife.
NEVER wear elastic garters or hose that are not properly measured.
NEVER apply extreme hot or cold to your feet.
NEVER wear cut-out shoes or sandals.
NEVER apply strong antiseptics or chemicals to your feet.

DO use anti-fungal powder between toes daily.
DO wear shoes and socks whenever you can.
DO visit your podiatrist regularly.
DO trim your nails (using a file or nail clipper) straight across.

Courtesy of Monoject.

Points to Remember when Teaching the Diabetic Patient

1. know your subject (diabetes) and your technique (insulin injection) thoroughly
2. use words the patient understands
3. instruct on the basis that the patient knows nothing about diabetes and insulin injection
4. ask questions of the patient to see how much he is learning
5. choose a quiet time and private place for instruction
6. don't flood the patient with too many facts at once
7. use cassettes, booklets, and visual aids that can be used by the patient when the instruction period is over
8. instruct a family member at the same time

REVIEW

A. Multiple Choice (Select the Best Answer)

1. Endocrine glands are:
   a. sebaceous glands
   b. ductless glands
   c. active in females only
   d. active in males only
2. The pancreas is unique because:
   a. it is the master gland of the body
   b. it is actually two glands
   c. it is both exocrine and endocrine
   d. it is unaffected by tumors
3. The urine test for sugar and acetone is:
   a. not a good indicator of hyperglycemia in the aged
   b. as accurate as a glucose tolerance test
   c. requires that the patient be fasting from midnight
   d. is accurate if the patient is on a fat free diet
4. When teaching the geriatric diabetic, the nurse should:
   a. present a thorough explanation of carbohydrate metabolism
   b. concentrate on diet therapy
   c. concentrate on urine testing
   d. present fundamental and important facts after getting to know the patient, his patterns of living, his educational background and his limitations—if any

5. The geriatric diabetic is very susceptible to:
   a. headache
   b. skin infections
   c. hearing impairment
   d. gait problems

B. Matching Test (Match Column 1 with Column 2)

Column 1	Column 2
a. Diabinese	_____6. insulin deficiency
b. diabetic retinopathy	_____7. tingling, burning, numbness
c. hyperglycemia	_____8. oral hypoglycemic
d. hypoglycemia	_____9. capillary hemorrhages
e. neuropathy	_____10. give orange juice

C. Briefly Answer the Following Questions

1. What are the symptoms and treatment of acidosis?
2. Give four recommendations for diabetic foot care.
3. Name one advantage of U-100 insulin.
4. Name a drug that might interfere with diabetic control.
5. What is meant by food exchange system?

16

The Special Sense Organs

Objectives

After completing this chapter the student should be able to:

- better understand how aging affects the sense organs
- perform ear and eye irrigations correctly
- instill ear, eye, and nose drops correctly
- understand how hearing aids work and be able to help patients with them
- communicate and work effectively with visually handicapped and blind elderly patients
- insert, remove, and care for eye protheses
- apply compresses to the eyes; remove minor foreign bodies from the eyes.
- use the following words correctly

Vocabulary

The following words relate to the material in this chapter. Look up the ones you do not know or are not sure of.

auditory	hyperextend	presbyopia
cerumen	hyperopia	presbycusis
conjunctiva	lacrimal glands	prosthesis
debility	otosclerosis	ptosis
diplopia	photophobia	retina

Review of the Anatomy of the Ear

Structures and Functions

Pinna. This is the outer ear. It is made up of two parts: the auricle (flap) and the external auditory canal. These two parts trap sound waves.

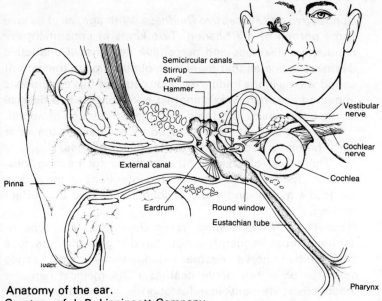

Anatomy of the ear.
Courtesy of J. B. Lippincott Company.

Middle Ear. This is separated from the external auditory canal by the tympanic membrane (eardrum). Three tiny, linked, but movable bones are located in the middle ear. They are the malleus (hammer), which is attached to the tympanic membrane, the incus (anvil), and the stapes (stirrup), attached to the inner ear. Sound waves from the air enter the external auditory canal, pass through the tympanic membrane, and cross the three bones to the inner ear.

Inner Ear. The inner ear transmits sounds to the brain. The chochlea, a complex, snail-like structure, is filled with a fluid that reacts to the vibrations of sound waves by rippling. The movement of the fluid activates the hair cells that make up the organ of Corti, where the hearing receptors are located. When these hair cells are stimulated, they send messages through the auditory nerve to the brain's center for hearing.

Age-Related Hearing Changes

1. *Conductive and Perceptive Deafness.* With age, all of us lose some portion of our hearing. Two kinds of impairment are conductive deafness and perceptive deafness. Conductive deafness indicates that there is an obstruction in the path of sound waves in the middle ear. One cause of this condition is impacted cerumen (wax); another is otosclerosis, a disease of the bone which interferes with the conduction of sound.

    Perceptive deafness is caused by a defect in the inner ear. The nerve endings just don't register sounds.

    There are, of course, other reasons for hearing loss, such as childhood injuries, repeated infections of the middle ear (otitis media) and acute childhood illnesses that affect hearing.

2. *Presbycusis (Degenerative Nerve Deafness).* The type of deafness most frequently encountered in geriatric nursing is degenerative nerve deafness (sometimes called senile deafness or eighth nerve deafness). Its medical name is presbycusis. Its early manifestation is an inability to hear high-frequency sounds. The condition is aggravated by

malnutrition, diabetes, circulatory disorders, and chronic systemic infections.

Presbycusis may lead to behavioral changes. The elderly patient may become irritable, depressed, and at times paranoid. He may withdraw and become isolated as he participates less and less in activities. It is difficult for him to use the telephone, a communication device we take for granted. It is estimated that one person in ten over the age of 65 has this problem.

3. *Impacted Cerumen.* The oil glands of the ear produce a wax called cerumen which, along with the hairs near the external opening, helps prevent foreign substances from entering the ear. Some individuals produce more cerumen than others and it can become hardened. A nurse or physician skilled in the procedure of removing earwax may be consulted. The patient should be cautioned, of course, against introducing anything into the ear to take out the wax because this only packs it more tightly against the eardrum. In addition, the eardrum could be punctured by using such objects as bobby pins, cotton tipped applicators, and so on.

Nursing Measures and Procedures

Helping with the Hearing Aid *

Being hard of hearing is serious, but not hopeless. There *are* corrective measures. First of all, the hard of hearing should see an otologist, a physician who specializes in diseases of the ear. If medication or surgery are not the answer, a hearing aid may be recommended. The nurse should know that such a device must be individually fitted and that the patient must be taught how to use and care for it. The following hints are written for differing degrees and types of losses. They will alert caregivers to the prob-

* This section (pages 299-306) is from Orientation to Hearing Aids by Gauger, J.S., Clymer, E.W., Young, M., and Woolever, L.D., National Technical Institute for the Deaf, Rochester Institute of Technology, Rochester, N.Y. 1978. These materials are available from: Alexander Graham Bell Association for the Deaf, Inc., 3417 Volta Place N.W., Washington, DC 20007.

lems that the hard of hearing older person may encounter with his hearing aid.

Initial Hearing Aid Use

1. A hearing aid should be used in quiet, familiar situations at first. It takes time for most persons to become adjusted to listening to amplified sounds. Gradually, use the aid in more difficult situations, such as large groups of people, large rooms, and noisy places such as restaurants. Success depends on the specific type and degree of loss a person has.

2. New hearing aid users should initiate use gradually. The skin which lines the ear canal is sensitive and, if irritated, takes time to heal.

3. A hearing aid has a volume control that has to be adjusted to different listening situations. Too little volume will cause other persons to have to speak louder than normal and too much volume will distort incoming sounds and over-amplify unwanted background sounds.

4. Anticipate that in everyday situations unexpected loud sounds can occur before the volume can be controlled. The user shouldn't become alarmed when this happens.

5. Some aids have tone control. Depending on the kind of hearing loss a person has, tone controls can markedly affect the clarity of speech which is heard with the hearing aid.

6. It takes time and practice to adjust to a new hearing aid. Several trips to the hearing aid dealer may be necessary in order to insure a properly fitted earmold.

Part-Time Hearing Aid Use (for Persons with a Mild Degree of Hearing Loss)

1. It may be that amplification is needed in certain types of situations only.

2. Hearing aids may hinder, rather than help, the communication of a person with a mild loss in some cases, particularly in noisy situations.

3. If part-time hearing aid use has been recommended, there is no logical reason to wear it in situations where it has not been found to be helpful.

Limitations of Hearing Aids

1.   A hearing aid is a mechanical prosthesis. It does not give normal hearing. It makes sounds and words *louder,* but it cannot make them *clearer* than a person's ability to understand speech clearly.

2.   While hearing aids have been constructed to provide a range of pitches or frequencies, they don't cover all the pitches the human ear is capable of hearing. For understanding speech, however, the hearing aid is adequate.

Common Complaints of Hearing Aid Users

1.   If the user's own voice sounds different or loud, it might be because:
   • he is very close to the microphone of the hearing aid, which picks up the sound and so his voice will sound louder than the voice of a person several feet away
   • a person with hearing loss isn't used to hearing his own voice so loud; sound is amplified and he is actually amplifying his own voice
   • hearing one's own voice through a mechanical instrument isn't the same as hearing it otherwise

2.   If the hearing aid seems to pick up more noise than speech:
   • turning the volume down may help
   • less volume will moderate background noise and voices will be heard better because people tend to speak louder when in noisy places

3.   A hearing aid that whistles:
   • may have a mechanical defect; it is possible to have sounds that come into the ear canal leak out and then feed back into the microphone, which causes a squeal; this may have to be investigated by the dealer
   • may have an improperly fitted earmold; this is the most common cause of squeals and whistles

4.   Improved hearing but no change in being able to understand may be due to:
   • lack of understanding of what a hearing aid can do, i.e., that it amplifies sound but does not make speech clearer
   • difficulty in being able to distinguish between vowel and consonental elements of speech; person will have to rely

on visual clues as well as the hearing aid to have maximum communication
- outside possibility that the hearing aid is faulty and should be checked

5. If wind whistles in the aid when outside or driving in a car with the window open:
- placing a small bit of porous material over the microphone may help
- this complaint is only of hearing aids worn on the head; a body model hearing aid is shielded by clothing.

6. Clothing noise (clothing rubbing on a body model hearing aid):
- not easily corrected; a harness that holds the aid may help
- unstarched clothing may help

7. If there is a feeling of "fullness" in the ear (common with new hearing aids):
- air may be trapped between the tips of the earmold and the drum membrane; usually passes in a few days
- dealer may have to "vent" the mold, but this may reduce clarity of speech

Suggestions for Some Specific Listening Situations

Hearing in Groups. It is extremely difficult to engage in group conversation when one is wearing a hearing aid. The criss-crossing of talk results in word scrambling. Keen concentration and attention is required. A beginning user should avoid group conversations. Later he should try groups but concentrate on one person at a time. The ability to concentrate in groups will develop in time.

Listening to Radio and TV. Announcers and commentators speak rapidly because of limited time allotments. The voices and sounds that are broadcast are mechanically reproduced and sometimes that results in poor quality. With practice, especially by paying attention to TV's visual clues, the person with a hearing aid can enjoy TV and also radio.

Using the Telephone. Many persons with even moderate to severe loss have little difficulty on the phone, especially if the telephone company has installed an amplifier. Those persons with poor ability to discriminate between speech sounds may have considerable difficulty.

The receiver should be held close to the microphone on the hearing aid. If the aid has a telephone pick-up switch, the switch should be flipped to "T" before the telephone is used. If a person is using a body hearing aid, he should hold the telephone upside down so the receiver is held close to the microphone on the body. The other end is help up to the mouth to speak into.

If hearing loss is not too severe in the unaided ear, it may be more practical to have the phone company install an amplifier which can be controlled for loudness by the speaker.

Sources for Help

If you need to find out more about hearing aids, contact the local Easter Seal Society, The American Hearing Society, or community speech and hearing center (see Appendix A). If necessary services are not offered locally, these agencies would be able to direct you to an appropriate source.

Care of the New Hearing Aid

Earmolds

Keep the earmold clean. Check it every day to be sure wax is not accumulating in the canal tip. If the opening is plugged with wax, simply remove it with a toothpick or pin. Detach it often and wash it with warm water and soap. Accumulations of wax on the outside can cause a poorly fitting mold and will result in feedback when the aid is turned on. *Do not* use alcohol to clean the mold as this has a tendency to cause cracks in the material.

Whistling or feedback is annoying. Be sure to check that the user knows how to put the earpiece in properly. The noises may be caused by a poorly fitting earpiece or by wax on the mold. Minor adjustments may have to be made by the dealer.

Earmolds need to be replaced periodically. Some types of materials will shrink over a period of time as they are exposed to the air. Persons' ears change in size (especially very young ears). But it's a mistake to think that there is no change in the size of the ear canal after maturity.

Tubing

The tubing which connects the hearing aid to the earmold will also need to be replaced periodically. It will dry out and have a tendency to crack. This is a very inexpensive part of the aid.

Batteries

If the hearing aid "goes dead" quickly, it is very likely the battery is no longer functioning. Replace it with a fresh one. Most hearing aids operate with mercury or silver oxide batteries. The voltage keeps a fairly stable level throughout its life, but will burn out quickly.

Some new batteries are defective. If a user puts a fresh battery in a hearing aid and it "warbles," it may be caused by a defective battery. Faulty batteries will be replaced free of charge.

Store batteries in a cool, dry place away from the direct rays of the sun or heat from a radiator. Don't keep too many on hand. Though the shelf life of mercury and silver oxide batteries is good, batteries which are stored six months or more may lose a good deal of their voltage and usefulness. It is better to buy only a half a dozen at a time and insure having fresh ones.

Avoid mixing old, worn-out batteries with a fresh supply. Since they "go out" rather quickly, always carry a spare for emergency use. Do not carry batteries loosely in a pocket. A plastic container protects better than a metal container.

Keep contacts clean. Oxygen in the air may cause corrosion on the metal contacts in the hearing aid or on the surface of the batteries, resulting in an unpleasant "frying" noise. If this occurs, the rubber eraser on the end of a lead pencil may be used to polish the contacts.

Cleaning and Repairs

A hearing aid needs to be cleaned periodically — about once a year. If the aid is exposed to an excessive amount of dirt, it can be done oftener.

Precautions

Do not drop the hearing aid. It is delicate and although it will take a considerable amount of jarring, the less there is the longer will be the lifetime of the aid.

Do not get the instrument wet.

Turn off aid when not in use to preserve battery.

First Aid for Hearing Aids

1. If the hearing aid gives no sound at all:
   Check the battery by trying a fresh one.
   The battery may be upside down.
   Check the earmold to be sure wax is not stopping up the opening.
   Check the tubing to see that it is not cracked, warped, or bent.
   If hearing aid has a telephone pick-up, be sure to check the switch; it may accidentally have been pushed to telephone.
   With a body aid, try a spare cord; the old one may have cracked or broken.
2. If the sounds are weaker than usual:
   Try the same things as above; especially try a new battery.
   A hearing aid exposed to excessively cold weather will be weak; it will act normally as soon as the indoor temperature takes effect.
3. If there are scratchy noises and if operation is intermittent:
   Clean battery and battery contact springs with a pencil eraser.
   Try a spare cord if it is a body aid.
   Move all switches back and forth; this may remove fine particles of lint or dust that can interfere with proper electrical contacts. Removing and inserting the cord plugs several times in the receiver may also correct the trouble.
4. If there are whistling noises:
   All hearing aid users are familiar with the "whistling" problem. If the aid does not whistle when it is removed from the ear with the volume turned up, the instrument isn't performing properly. Feedback can be caused by certain condi-

tions existing inside the instrument. A leak between any connections from the aid to the earmold can cause feedback.

Replacing the Hearing Aid

A hearing aid does not last indefinitely, nor does any mechanical device. The average length of time during which an aid will perform satisfactorily is from four to six years. Some people have them for ten years. An aid can be changed for a new model, just like a car. Of course, a great deal depends on the care which is given to the aid, but every aid will wear out sooner or later. If costly repairs are needed, it may be time to replace the aid.

Irrigating the Ear and Instilling Medications

There is an important difference between ear irrigations and ear instillations. An irrigation is a solution that flows over a specific area. An instillation is the topical administration of a drug drop by drop to a specific site that will benefit by the action of the drug being instilled.

Ear irrigations are used to remove impacted cerumen, the protective secretion produced by glands in the ear. The production of cerumen may increase when the ear is infected by fungi or bacteria. Dark-haired people produce more cerumen than light-haired people.

If cerumen becomes hard and impacted it will impair hearing and may cause discomfort. Instilling hydrogen peroxide half an hour before the irrigation helps to soften the ear wax. In stubborn cases, drops of mineral oil should be instilled several days before irrigation.

Equipment
hydrogen peroxide

rubber bulb syringe or

    metal Pomeroy syringe

towel

dropper

curved basin

protective underpad

prescribed solution

Sequence
1. identify and screen patient; explain procedure to him
2. ask patient to turn head to side with affected ear uppermost

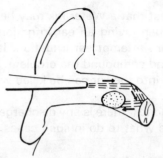

Ear irrigation. Courtesy of W. B. Saunders Company.

3. pull the ear upward and backward in order to straighten the normally curved auditory canal
4. instill a few drops of hydrogen peroxide in the ear; tell patient to hold this position for 10 or 15 minutes and reassure patient that the bubbling and fizzing is the sound that hydrogen peroxide normally makes
5. return to patient to complete procedure; place curved basin under the ear to be irrigated; have patient hold this to catch return flow
6. drape patient with protective pad and towel
7. fill syringe with solution at tepid temperature (check doctor's order before beginning procedure for prescribed solution.)
8. pull the outer ear upward and backward
9. direct the flow of solution toward the side of the auditory canal, *not* toward the center of the canal (to avoid pushing the impaction against the eardrum); administer solution slowly
10. watch for wax returns; stop irrigation when plug of cerumen is noted in returns
11. aftercare of patient as needed; watch for dizziness
12. record results and note how patient tolerated procedure

Abbreviations Used for Ear Treatments and Medications

A.D.	aurio dextra	right ear
A.S.	aurio sinestra	left ear
A.U.	aures utrae	both ears

NOTES: Some texts suggest that a Water Pik may be used successfully at low pressure when giving an ear irrigation. If a foreign body is in the ear, *do not* attempt ear irrigation. It may cause the obstruction to swell and compound the problem. See a physician. Bugs that fly or crawl into the ear can be killed with oil instillation and then flushed out.

Ear irrigation should not be done if there is any discharge from the ear. Let the physician decide what to do in such cases.

A Review of Terminology Relating to the Ear

audiometer—instrument used to measure hearing ability

myringotomy—surgical incision of the tympanic membrane to allow drainage

otoscope—instrument used to examine external auditory canal

otologist—physician who specializes in ear diseases

tinnitus—sensation of ringing in the ears

vertigo—dizziness; characteristic of Meniere's syndrome, a disturbance of the semicircular canals in the inner ear (which aid in maintaining body balance); may eventually lead to deafness

Anatomy of the Eye

The eyeball is made up of three layers of tissues:

Sclera. This is the tough outer layer. It serves as a supporting framework for the two inner layers. Light enters through the transparent cornea in front of the eye and the aqueous humor (clear fluied) lies right behind the cornea.

Middle Layer. This is divided into three parts: the choroid, which contains blood vessels; the ciliary body, which contains the ciliary muscles that keep the lens in place; and the iris, the colored part of the eye.

Retina. This is the inner layer of the eyeball. It has light sensitive cells (rods and cones) and touches the choroid. Nerve fibers in front of the rods and cones mesh to form the optic nerve.

The eyeball is protected by the bony orbit in which it lies. Also contributing to protection are the eye lashes, lids, and brows.

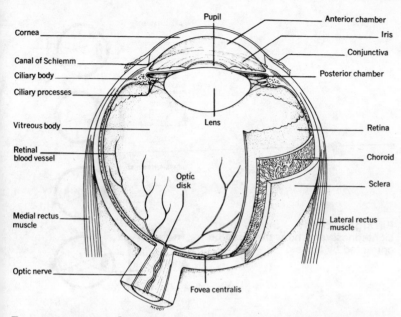

Transverse section of the eye. Courtesy of J. B. Lippincott Company.

Light rays are slightly bent toward each other as they meet the cornea. The iris regulates the amount of light that enters the eye because it is able to change the size of the pupil. The pupil contracts if too much light is beamed toward the eye, and it expands if light is dim. The rays bend even more as they pass through the curved lens. They meet at the focus which *should* be on the retina. Light rays will be blurred if they meet in *front* of or in *back* of the retina. The eye is constructed so we can focus perfectly on near or far objects—but not simultaneously. Light enters the eye and changes a chemical in the retina which permits us to see.

If an eyeball is too long, the lens brings the light rays into focus too far in front of the retina. Concave lenses are used to compensate for this nearsightedness.

Farsightedness occurs when the eyeball is too short and rays focus *behind* the retina. Glasses with convex lenses help sharpen vision.

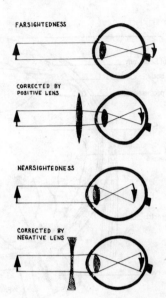

Farsightedness and near-sightedness and how they can be corrected by lenses.

Age-Related Visual Changes

1. *Slowed Responses.* The slowed responses to stimuli that are noticeable in so many elderly patients' reactions is also true of the eye. The slowness with which the eye reacts to dust specks and other foreign bodies makes it vulnerable to injury.

2. *Reduced Secretions.* The tear-producing lacrimal glands secrete less fluid, and therefore the eyes look dry and lack luster.

3. *Diminished Visual Perception, Ulcers, Iritis.* Visual perception diminishes for several reasons. There is a degeneration of the blood vessels that nourish the tissues; the pupil is smaller and less light gets to the retina. Ulcers of the cornea and inflammation of the iris (iritis) occur frequently, and just as frequently the elderly person puts off seeking treatment, attributing many of these changes to "old age."

4. *Detached Retina.* This condition is often found in the elderly since chronic disease, old age, and debility

predispose to this problem, in which the retina separates from the choroid. Trauma can also cause this condition, as in the case of a severe shaking up, with or without bruises, and other injuri s from accidents. A detached retina can be treated surgically, but the condition sometimes recurs. Strict attention to postoperative measures and positive health practices during convalescence help prevent recurrences.

5. *Corneal Ulcers.* These occur following fever, nutritional deficiencies, or a stroke. They can also be caused by irritation, as from eyelashes. Reduced muscle tone and loss of elasticity of the skin cause ectropion, the turning outward of the lower eyelid, and entropion, a turning inward of the upper eyelid. Entropion irritation can cause corneal ulcers because the lashes can scratch the cornea. Ectropion exposes the conjunctiva in the lower lid and dries the natural secretions before they are able to lubricate the cornea.

6. *Glaucoma.* Glaucoma, a disease characterized by increased intraocular pressure, causes blindness in many elderly. Some early symptoms are: headache, loss of peripheral vision, and seeing halos around lights. Glaucoma is never cured, although treatment relieves symptoms. While physician's orders are specific, there are some general guidelines nurses should know when caring for patients with glaucoma. Increased intraocular pressure can result from stress, wearing tight clothing, upper respiratory infections, and excessive fluids. Activities to be encouraged are moderation in exercise and in using the eyes, avoiding constipation, and use of medications with the physician's authority *only*. The patient should wear a Medic-alert bracelet which identifies him as having glaucoma.

7. *Cataracts.* This condition, in which the lens becomes clouded, is very common among the elderly. About eight out of ten geriatric patients 80 and over have some loss of the transparency of the lens. The cause of senile cataracts is unknown. Fortunately, surgery for this problem is highly successful, restoring vision in 95 percent of those patients who have uncomplicated cataracts.

8. *Blindness.* Blindness can occur when nephritis with high blood pressure is present in the geriatric patient. Diabetic retinopathy, caused by hemorrhaging of the small blood vessels that nourish the retina, causes blindness in young as well as old persons.

9. *Presbyopia.* Even if the aged adult is in excellent health with no eye pathology, there are vision changes he probably can't avoid. The most common of these is presbyopia (farsightedness), a condition caused by the decreasing elasticity of the lens, which results in a lack of accommodation for near vision. A prescription for reading glasses corrects this deficiency. This decreasing elasticity begins at about the age of 45.

Nursing Measures and Procedures for Caring for the Eyes

The nurse can be helpful by discouraging people from using glasses that are not specifically prescribed for them. Many elderly women take better care of their hair, and many elderly men take better care of their cars than of their eyes. It's common practice not only to borrow eyeglasses but also to use outdated eye medications, or eye medications that are prescribed for someone else.

Another drawback to maintaining optimum eye care is the tendency to put off seeing a physician when there are unpleasant symptoms with either the fear that "if I go, he'll find something wrong," or "maybe things will clear up in a few days."

Many people don't differentiate between an optician, an optometrist and an ophthalmologist. An optician grinds and fits lenses; an optometrist is a nonmedical person who examines, prescribes, and adjusts lenses; and an ophthalmologist is a physician trained in diagnosing and treating diseases of the eye.

Care of the eyes and of eyesight includes good nutritional intake. For example, night blindness (absent or defective vision in the dark) may result from a vitamin A deficiency as well as from degenerative changes of the aging adult. Diet may not be able to cure eye diseases but a balanced diet certainly can delay aging's unpleasant side effects by slowing lens opacity and probably deterring many other degenerative processes.

Suggestions for Working with the Visually Handicapped*

1. Provide adequate lighting at all times, especially for reading, sewing, writing, and similar activities. Lighting is extremely important. A room that is well lit is better than a room that has only a table lamp or floor lamp. The reason is that it is hard for an elderly person to adapt from light to dark and vice versa. A lamp accentuates light in a small area with vast areas of darkness around it. It's hard to accommodate to this if you're over 65.

2. Avoid bright glare, e.g., highly polished floors, windows without curtains or shades.

3. Supply a nightlight in the bathroom, kitchen or any other area where the individual is likely to go at night.

4. Elderly people should be discouraged from driving at night because of "night blindness."

5. Large-print newspapers, magazines, and books should be made available.

6. Take advantage of other useful aids that are available such as needle threaders and playing cards with enlarged figures and numbers.

7. Talking book records and machines can be obtained free from the Library of Congress.

8. Face the visually handicapped person when speaking to him.

9. It is easier for a visually impaired person to lipread if the speaker wears bright lipstick.

10. Do not cover your mouth, smoke, or chew gum when speaking to a visually handicapped person.

11. Provide a transistor radio for the handicapped person to carry from place to place.

12. Special dials for phones are available which enlarge the numbers and glow in the dark; provide if possible.

* Courtesy of Holyoke Geriatric Convalescent Center, Holyoke, Mass.

13. Do not move furniture or belongings around without explaining what you are doing and why.
14. Give simple but detailed instructions for anything you plan to do. Wheelchair patients in particular need to be told about obstacles, warned that they will be pulled backwards, and so on, to diminish their fears.
15. Large clocks and large calendars are a must for orientation.
16. Do not use colors that blend. For example, avoid white dishes on a white table, beige light switches on beige walls, and so on.
17. Eyeglasses must be cleaned often and checked for scratched lenses, cracks, or faulty screws. Eyes should be checked regularly.

Suggestions for Working with Blind Elders*
1. Face the person directly when speaking to him.
2. Touch the person you're speaking to: a handshake will help him place where you are. It's especially important to touch hallucinating patients when speaking to them. However, be sure to speak before touching a blind person.
3. Provide pockets on clothing.
4. Provide a transistor radio.
5. A rope or cord leading to the bathroom may be useful. Be careful that it doesn't create a hazard, however.
6. Do not move personal belongings or furniture around.
7. Remove the glass from clocks so the person can tell time by touch. Have him use a Braille wristwatch.
8. Provide a calendar with raised letters and numbers.
9. Arrange for free talking books from the Library of Congress.
10. Speak clearly, slowly, and distinctly. If the person is confused or has a short attention span, allow for this.
11. Check to see if the person's hearing is impaired also. You may have to move closer or talk directly into his ear.
12. Give the blind person simple but detailed instructions about all the things you plan to do to him. Remember that there are no nonverbal or visual clues to help the person understand. It

* *Courtesy of Holyoke Geriatric Convalescent Center, Holyoke, Massachusetts.*

is especially important to explain to the blind person what is happening in group meetings.

13. Do not leave an elderly blind person alone in his room for long periods of time. He may begin to hallucinate.

14. Do not change the daily schedule. Elderly people often judge the time of day by the day's regular events; they do not have sunrise and sunset for reminders.

15. Use as many external clues as possible, e.g., clocks that chime, a noon whistle, intercom, radio, and so on.

16. Constantly use sensory stimulation through touch, sounds, and smells since visual stimulation is absent. Increase such stimulation if there are signs of apathy, withdrawal, depression, or a diagnosis of chronic brain syndrome.

17. The newly blinded individual should be told about his disability in a straightforward manner. It decreases the impact of the disability.

Instillation of Eye Medications

For instillation, the patient may be in bed or seated in a chair. Any solution or ointment instilled should be sterile and used for the individual patient only. Most eye drops have the dropper built

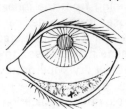

Eye drops are administered into the lower fornix (indicated by X). Courtesy of W. B. Saunders.

into the bottle cap, but there may be times when the nurse will use a sterile eye dropper. As the drops are instilled, the nurse should be careful to drop the solution into the lower conjunctival sac (in the lower eyelid) to avoid traumatizing the sensitive cornea. The medication is recorded after the procedure by indicating the treated eye as follows:

O · D ·	oculus dexter	right eye
O · S ·	oculus sinister	left eye
O · U ·	oculo utro	both eyes

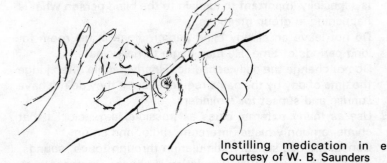

Instilling medication in eye
Courtesy of W. B. Saunders

Equipment
medication
sterile eye dropper, if needed
sterile cotton balls or gauze squares

Sequence
1. identify patient; introduce self; explain procedure; screen patient
2. with cotton ball or gauze square cleanse the affected eye, wiping from the inner canthus (corner of the eye near the nose) to the outer canthus; if there is a discharge from the eye, or if it is encrusted with dried secretions, sterile normal saline may be used to cleanse the affected eye
3. with a dry wipe protecting the finger of the nurse, depress the eyelid, tell the patient to look upward, and drop the prescribed medication into the lower conjunctival sac to avoid traumatizing the sensitive cornea.
4. caution the patient not to rub the eye; rather, suggest he close both eyes and move them around to help distribute the medication
5. record the time, amount of drug, patient's reaction, and which eye was treated

NOTES: If an eye ointment is to be applied, follow the same basic procedure but apply a thin line of the ointment along the conjunctiva of the lower lid.

Naturally, the nurse will wash her hands thoroughly *before* giving eye medications; this includes handwashing after treating *each* eye if both eyes are medicated in order to avoid cross contamination. The nurse should again wash her hands *after* the procedure is concluded.

Eye Irrigation

Purposes
to cleanse the eyes
to treat for inflammation, and so on

Equipment

prescribed solution, tepid temperature	curved basin
	towel
rubber bulb syringe or eye dropper as ordered	waterproof protective pad
	gauze squares

Sequence
1. identify patient; introduce self; explain procedure; screen patient
2. have patient tip head toward the *affected* side so solution flows from inner aspect of eye to outer (to avoid cross contamination)
3. place protective underpad and towel over shoulder, tuck up under head and neck so gown and sheets aren't saturated
4. have patient hold curved basin at cheek on affected side to catch waste solution
5. depress lower conjunctival sac while holding upper lid open
6. gently introduce tepid solution from the inner canthus toward the outer canthus, being careful not to touch the eye, eyelid, or eyelashes with the tip of dropper or syringe; allow patient to blink from time to time
7. after prescribed length of time for treatment, have patient close eyes; blot dry
8. record as for instillation

Removal of a Foreign Body
Eyes are self-cleansing and the use of over-the-counter eye-cleansing preparations for the geriatric patient should be discouraged. Valuable time is lost with such self-medication. Many a physician has struggled to conceal his frustration when faced with a health problem that could have been solved quickly and easily if only the patient turned up in his office sooner.

Occasionally the nurse will be asked to remove a foreign body from the eye. Of course, anything other than a small dirt particle or an eyelash should be referred to a physician.

Sequence
1. wash hands
2. grasp upper lid by the lashes and pull outward and downward; the eye will tear and may wash out the foreign body
3. evert upper lid on an applicator
4. holding the eyelid everted, slide the applicator out
5. remove lash or cinder with applicator

Compresses
Hot or cold eye compresses may be ordered. The important aspect of using compresses is to avoid cross-contamination. This means that either the nurse will use sterile gloves and surgical aseptic technique or she will use gauze-wrapped tongue blades that have been sterilized, being careful to handle them by the wooden end. Sometimes a layer of sterile Vaseline is applied to protect the lid before the compress is administered. This should be stated in the physician's order.

Care of the Eye Prosthesis
An enucleation, removal of an eye, is surgery performed in case of malignancy or severe eye trauma. A solid ballshaped implant can be attached to the eye muscles. After healing is complete, a glass or plastic prosthesis can be fitted over the implant. This operation permits the prosthesis to move as the healthy eye focuses.

Most patients in this situation care for their own prosthesis, but occasionally the nurse assists.

NOTE: Scrupulous cleanliness of the eye and of the socket are necessary to prevent infections and irrigations. The prosthesis should be gently cleansed with warm water and mild soap or saline. It should be stored in a suitable place. Generally, the eye is kept in water if it is not being worn.

Insertion of an Artificial Eye

1.   wash hands before handling an artificial eye and before touching the socket
2.   rinse prosthesis with saline or with water; sometimes the physician's order may require the socket to be rinsed also
3.   hold the eye so that the pointed end is toward the nose
4.   lift the upper lid and slide the eye under the lid
5.   hold the eye in place, pull the lower lid down until it slides over the lower edge of the eye

Removal of an Artificial Eye

1.   wash hands
2.   depress the lower lid
3.   cup hand under the eye
4.   exert slight pressure under the eye; it will slip out

NOTE: Artificial eyes are fragile and should be inserted and removed while the patient is leaning over a bed or a pillow.

Terminology Relating to the Eye

blepharitis—inflammation of the edges of the eyelid

cocaine hydrochloride—local anesthetic used on cornea when removing foreign bodies

keratitis—inflammation of the cornea

myotic—drug that contracts the pupil; used to reduce intra-ocular pressure in glaucoma (example: pilocarpine nitrate)

mydriatic—drug instilled to dilate pupils (example: atropine sulfate)

ophthalmoscope—instrument used to visualize the vitreous body, optic disk, retinal arteries and veins

strabismus—squint; cross-eye

sty —infection on the edge of the eyelid

tonometer—specially designed instrument that rests on the eyeball and is used to determine the intraocular pressure of the eyeball

uveitis—inflammation of the ciliary body, iris, choroid

Taste and Smell

Taste buds are located primarily on the surface of the tongue and in three places in the throat. Many substances taken into the mouth cause the taste buds to produce the sensation of taste. It's not clearly known how this happens.

The organ of smell is the nose. As we breathe, we inhale odorous gases that are mixed with the natural gases of the air. These gases touch a small cluster of epithelial cells that line the upper part of the inner surface of the nose. The cells then generate impulses that race along a pair of nerves to the cerebrum where the interpretation is an odor. Every gas we inhale does not set up the ''smell'' sensation. However, the more of an odorous gas that does contact these special cells, the stronger the odor.

The sense of smell can weaken. That's why it's possible to enter a room, smell a strong odor, and after a while barely notice it.

Excessive mucus secretion can mask the sense of smell. If one has a cold, mucus coats the epithelial cells that pick up scent and inhibits gases from contacting them.

Age-Related Changes in Taste and Smell

Impaired smell among the elderly is common. It can actually be a safety hazard, as in the case of fire, escaping gas, or spoiled food.

The senses of smell and taste are linked. If something smells good we are inclined to taste it. The decline in appetite noticed in many geriatric patients is partly because of loss of smell and partly because there is a marked decrease in taste buds. By the age of 75, 65 percent of the taste buds are lost.

Dietitians in nursing homes and hospitals and other health care workers seem to feel that elderly adults prefer bland food. They don't. They like highly seasoned food because it takes more sugar to get the right sweet taste and more of other seasonings to make foods palatable. It is true, of course, that many of the elderly are on bland diets because of medical or surgical problems, but those who aren't should be allowed condiments.

The elderly like variety but the variety should include familiar foods because that's what their digestive tracts are used to. Long periods of time between meals should be avoided. Five or six small meals a day are preferable to three large meals.

Nursing Measure

Nose Drop Instillation

Nose drops are drugs that are made up in solutions of normal saline. Oily solutions are never used because of the danger of aspiration pneumonia.

To administer nose drops, ask the patient to sit with his head and neck hyperextended. If the patient is confined to bed, his head may be tilted back over a pillow. The solutions should flow to the back of the nose. Before giving nose drops, the patient may gently blow both nostrils together to clear the nose.

The tip of the dropper is placed just inside the nose and the prescribed medication instilled. The patient should maintain his position for several minutes after the instillation. If the solution runs down the back of the throat, the patient will want to expectorate, so tissues should be provided. He should be encouraged not to blow his nose for half an hour after the instillation.

REVIEW

A. Multiple Choice (Select the Best Answer)

1. The middle ear is separated from the external auditory canal by:
   a. the cochlea
   b. the organ of Corti
   c. the tympanic membrane
   d. the malleus

2. The type of deafness the geriatric nurse most frequently encounters is:
   a. presbycusis
   b. conductive nerve deafness
   c. otosclerosis
   d. impacted cerumen

3. Impacted cerumen may be softened with:
   a. moistened q tips
   b. Dobell's solution
   c. hydrogen peroxide
   d. sterile water

4. Light sensitive cells are:
   a. ciliary bodies
   b. rods and cones
   c. neurons
   d. electrons

5. Farsightedness occurs when:
   a. light rays focus too far in front of the retina
   b. light rays fail to be regulated by the iris
   c. light rays fail to be regulated by the choroid
   d. light rays focus too far behind the retina

B. Matching Test (Match Column 1 with Column 2)

Column 1	Column 2
a. Meniere's syndrome	_____6. increased intraocular pressure
b. myringotomy	_____7. clouding of lens
c. tinnitus	_____8. surgical opening into tympanic membrane
d. glaucoma	_____9. ringing in ears
e. cataract	_____10. vertigo

C. Briefly Answer the Following Questions

1. Why does visual perception diminish with age?
2. What other problems aggravate presbycusis?
3. Describe the differences between an optician, an optometrist and an ophthalmologist.
4. Explain the difference between an instillation and an irrigation.
5. Why is there a decline in the appetite of the geriatric patient?

References

Chapters 1, 2, and 3

Abernathy, J. B., *Old Is Not a Four-Letter Word.* Abingdon Press, Nashville, 1975

American Nursing Home Association, *Thinking About a Nursing Home?* ANHA Pub. 0773-2

Blazer, Dan, "Techniques for Communicating With Your Elderly Patient." *Geriatrics,* Nov. 1978, p. 79

Burnside, I., *Psychosocial Nursing Care of the Aged.* McGraw-Hill, New York, 1973

Butler, R. N. and Lewis, M. I., *Aging and Mental Health.* Mosby, St. Louis, 1978

Curtain, S., *Nobody Ever Died of Old Age.* Little, Brown, Boston, 1972

Diekelmann, Nancy, *Primary Health Care of the Well Adult.* New York: McGraw-Hill, 1977

Eliopoulos, C., *Gerontological Nursing.* Harper and Row, New York, 1979

Larkin, Jon A., "Brandywine House: A Communal Living Experiment." *Perspective on Aging,* March/April, 1978

Linden, M. E., *Retirement and the Elderly: Problems and Practical Therapy.* (scientific exhibit) American Geriatrics Society, April 16-17 1975

Stevens, C. B., *Special Needs of Long Term Patients.* Lippincott, Philadelphia, 1974

Chapters 4 and 5

American Heart Association, *Aphasia and the Family.* New York, 1974

Butler, R., and Lewis, M., *Aging and Mental Health.* C.V. Mosby, St. Louis, 1977

Butler, R. N., *Why Survive? Being Old in America.* Harper and Row, New York, 1975

Gage, F., "Suicide in the Aged." *American Journal of Nursing,* 71 (11): 2153-2155, November, 1971

Goldfarb, A. I., *Aging and Organic Brain Syndrome.* Health Learning Systems Inc., 1-22, 1974

Gordon, S. K., "The Phenomenon of Depression in Old Age." *Gerontologist,* 13 (1): 100-105, Spring, 1973

King, M. S., "Drugs, Drinking and the Elderly." *The Boston Globe,* June 29, 1979, p. 23

Linden, Maurice E., "Retirement and the Elderly Patient." Address at American Geriatrics Society's 32nd annual meeting, Miami Beach, FL, 1975

Looney, D. S., "Senility Is also a State of Mind." *National Observer,* March 31, 1973, p. 1

Phillips, D. F., "Reality Orientation." *Journal of the American Hospital Association,* 47: 46-101, 1973

Saxon, S., and Etten, M., *Physical Change and Aging: A Guide for the Helping Professions.* Tiresias Press, New York, 1978

Taulbee, L., and Folsom, J., "Reality Orientation for Geriatric Patients." *Hospital and Community Psychiatry,* 17:133-135, 1966

Whitehead, J. M., *Psychiatric Disorders in Old Age.* Springer, New York, 1974

Chapter 6

Friedeman, Joyce S., "Sexuality in Older Persons: Implications for Nursing Practice." *Nursing Forum,* 1979 (18:1): 92-101

Griggs, Winona, "Staying Well While Growing Old . . . Sex and the Elderly." *AJN* 78(8): 1352-1354

Masters, William H. and Johnson, Virginia E., *Human Sexual Response,* Little, Brown and Co., 1966, pp. 238-240

Stanford, Dennyse, "All About Sex . . . . After Middle Age," *AJN* 77(4), pp. 608-611

Watts, Rosalyn J., "The Physiological Interrelationships between Depression, Drugs, and Sexuality." *Nursing Forum,* 1978 (17:2): 168-183

Chapter 7

Blackburn, G. L., et. al., "Nutritional and Metabolic Assessment of the Hospitalized Patient." *Journal of Parenteral and Enteral Nutrition* 1 (1): 11-22 January/February 1977

Grills, N. J., "Nutritional Needs of Elderly Women." *Clinical Obstetrics and Gynecology* 20 (1): 137-143 March 1977

Harrill, I., et al, "Observations on Food Acceptance By Elderly Women." *The Gerontologist* 16 (4): 394-399 August 1976

Klinger, J. L., et al., *Mealtime Manual for the Aged and Handicapped.* Institute of Rehabilitation Medicine, New York University Medical Center, Essandess Special Editions, New York, 1970

Lasson, R., "Do Nutritional Needs Change With Age?" *Retirement Living* 13 (11): p. 21 November 1973

Lewis, Clara, *Nutritional Considerations for the Elderly*. F.A. Davis Philadelphia, 1978

Lipton, M. A., "Nutritional Fads and the Search for Mental Health." University of North Carolina, Bulletin 21 (Autumn issue) 4-10, 1975

Mayer, Jean, *Human Nutrition*. Charles C. Thomas, Springfield, 1974

Mayo Clinic Diet Manual. W. B. Saunders, Philadelphia, 1971

Mercer, M., "The Health Risk Older People Ignore." *McCalls* 99 (11): 12-16, August, 1972

National Dairy Council: *To Your Health In Your Second Fifty Years*. 1974

Organ, C., Finn, M., "The Importance of Nutritional Support For the Elderly Surgical Patient." *Geriatrics* 32 (5): 77-84, May, 1977

Robinson, C. H., *Basic Nutrition and Diet Therapy*. Macmillan, New York, 1970

Rombauer, I., Becker, M., *The Joy of Cooking*. New American Library, New York, 1975

Ten-State Nutritional Survey, 1968-1970. Center for Disease Control Washington, D.C., 1972

Chapters 8 through 16

American Foundation for the Blind, *An Introduction to Working with the Aging Person Who Is Visually Handicapped*. New York, 1972

Anthony, Catherine P., *Structure and Function of the Body*. Mosby, St. Louis, 1976

Beland, Irene and Passos, Joyce, *Clinical Nursing: Pathophysiological and Psychosocial Approaches*. Macmillan, New York, 1975

Brunner, Lillian and Suddarth, Doris, *Textbook of Medical-Surgical Nursing*. Lippincott, Philadelphia, 1975

Burnside, I. M., "Clocks and Calendars." *American Journal of Nursing*, 70 (5): 117-119, January 1970

Caldwell, Esther and Hegner, Barbara, *Geriatric Nursing: A Study of Maturity*. Delmar, Albany, 1972

Diekelmann, Nancy, *Primary Health Care of the Well Adult*. McGraw-Hill, New York, 1977

Dison, Norma, *Clinical Nursing Techniques*. Mosby, Philadelphia, 1979

Eliopoulos, Charlotte, *Gerontological Nursing*. Harper and Row, New York 1979

Ferris, Elvira, and Skelley, Esther, *Body Structure and Functions*. Delmar Publishers, Albany, 1968

Freese, A. S., "If You Can't Hear." *Modern Maturity*, 22 (1): 31-32, February-March 1979

French, Ruth, *Guide to Diagnostic Procedures*. McGraw-Hill, New York, 1975

Harless, E. L. and Rupp R. R., "Aural Rehabilitation and the Elderly." *Journal of Speech and Hearing Disorders,* vol. 37 267-273, 1972

Hoffman, Claire, Lipkin, Gladys, and Thompson, Ella, *Simplified Nursing.* Lippincott, Philadelphia, 1968

Hole, John W., *Human Anatomy and Physiology.* Wm. C. Brown, Dubuque, 1978

Hornemann, Grace, *Basic Nursing Procedures.* Delmar, Albany, 1972

Keane, Claire Brackman, *Essentials of Nursing.* Saunders, Philadelphia, 1979

King, Eunice M. et al., *Illustrated Manual of Nursing Techniques.* Lippincott, Philadelphia, 1976

Lewis, Lu Verne Wolff, *Fundamental Skills in Patient Care.* Lippincott, Philadelphia, 1976

Macleod, John, ed., *Davidson's Principles and Practice of Medicine.* Churchill Livingstone, Edinburgh, 1975

Mason, Mildred A., *Basic Medical-Surgical Nursing.* Macmillan, New York, 1978

Mosby's *Comprehensive Review of Nursing.* Mosby, St. Louis, 1977

O'Brien, Maureen J., *The Care of the Aged: A Guide for the Licensed Practical Nurse.* Mosby, St. Louis, 1971

Ruch, Theodore C. and Patton, Harry D., *Physiology and Biophysics.* Saunders, London, 1974

Rupp, R. R., "Understanding the Problem of Presbycusis." *Geriatrics,* vol. 25, 100-107

Scherer, Jeanne C., *Introductory Medical-Surgical Nursing.* Lippincott, Philadelphia, 1977

Shaefer, Kathleen, *Medical Surgical Nursing.* Mosby, St. Louis, 1977

Smith, Dorothy W. and Hanley, Carol P., *Care of the Adult Patient: Medical-Surgical Nursing.* Lippincott, Philadelphia, 1975

Stevens, Marion, K., *Geriatric Nursing for Practical Nurses.* Saunders, Philadelphia, 1973

Sutton, Audrey Latshaw, *Bedside Nursing Techniques in Medicine and Surgery.* Saunders, Philadelphia, 1974

Thompson, Ella and Roedahl, Caroline, *Textbook of Basic Nursing.* Lippincott, Philadelphia, 1973

Watson, Jeannette E., *Medical-Surgical Nursing and Related Physiology.* Saunders, Philadelphia, 1972

Wolff, Lu Verne, et al., *Fundamentals of Nursing: The Humanities and the Sciences in Nursing.* Lippincott, Philadelphia, 1979

Van Ruper, C., *Speech Correction: Principles and Methods.* Prentice-Hall, Englewood-Cliffs, N.J., 1963

Ventura, F. P. "Counselling the Hearing Impaired Geriatric Patient." *Patient Counselling and Health Education,* 1 (1) 22-25, 1978

Verner, Lawrence, *Mathematics for Health Practitioners: Basic Concepts and Clinical Applications.* Lippincott, Philadelphia, 1978

Appendix

Organizations that Provide Information on Health Maintenance

American Association of Homes for the Aging
1050 17th Street N.W., Washington, DC   20036

American Association of Retired Persons
1225 Connecticut Avenue, N.W., Washington DC   20036

American Cancer Society
219 E. 42 Street, New York, NY   10017

American Diabetes Association
18 E. 48 Street, New York, NY   10017

American Foundation for the Blind
15 West 16 Street, New York, NY   10011

American Heart Association
7320 Greenville Avenue, Dallas, TX   75231

American Nursing Home Association
1200 15 Street, N.W., Washington DC   20005
(This association is dedicated to improving health care of the convalescent and chronically ill of all ages. It publishes a guide to selecting a nursing home titled *Thinking About a Nursing Home?* which is available by writing to the above address. The guide stresses that the type of facility selected depends on the needs of the individual, and that the family physician is usually the best one qualified to discuss those needs.)

American Occupational Therapy Association
6000 Executive Boulevard, Rockville, MD   20852

American Orthotics and Prosthetics Association
1440 N Street, N.W., Washington, DC   20005

American Physical Therapy Association
1156 15 Street, N.W., Washington, DC   20005
(For rehabilitation assistance.)

American Speech and Hearing Association
9030 Old Georgetown Road, N.W., Washington DC   20014

Arthritis Foundation
1212 Avenue of the Americas, New York, NY   10036

Institute of Rehabilitation Medicine
400 East 34 Street, New York, NY   10016

National Association for the Deaf (NAD)
814 Thayer Avenue, Silver Spring, MD   20910

National Association for Speech and Hearing Action (NASHA)
814 Thayer Avenue #102, Silver Spring, MD   20910
> (Advocate for community hearing and speech centers; focuses on consumer protection.)

National Council of Community Mental Health Centers
2502 Belmont Boulevard, Nashville, TN   37212

The National Council on the Aging
1828 L Street N.W., Washington, DC   20036
> The NCOA was established in 1950 and it is the leading national organization of professionals and volunteers involved in everything that affects the quality of life for older Americans. This organization seeks solutions to problems that include the provision of adequate medical care, housing employment, transportation and further education and training. It is a central national resource for research, planning, training, information projects, technical consultation and publications relating to older persons. The principal source of income for the NCOA is grants and contracts from the federal government, membership dues, sale of publications and individual contributions. Further information is available by writing to the above address.

National Easter Seal Society for Crippled Children and Adults
2023 West Ogden Avenue, Chicago, IL   60612

National Institute on Adult Day Care
c/o National Council on the Aging
1828 L Street N.W., Washington, DC   20036
> NIAD evolved from the National Task Force on Adult Day Care that was established within the National Council on the Aging in April, 1978. The NIAD recognizes the country's growing need for special programs for the elderly who are functionally disabled. Adult day care refers generically to a variety of programs, each a composite of services that range from social and health related to active rehabilitation and physical and mental health.

Older Americans Resources and Services
Duke University Medical Center, Box 3003, Durham, NC   27710

Special Services

Amplification for TV and telephones; alarm clocks for hearing impaired:

Hal-Hen Company
36-14 11 Street, Long Island, NY 11106

Televox Industries
6022 West Pico Boulevard, Los Angeles, CA 90035

For medical and nursing assistance:

local county medical society
local Visiting Nurses Association
local chapter of American Heart Association

COMMON ABBREVIATIONS

aa — of each	m. — minim
abd. — abdomen	mg. — milligram
a.c. — before meals	Mg — magnesium
ad lib — as much as desired	ml. — milliliter
AM — morning	N — nitrogen
amb. — ambulatory	Na — sodium
amt. — amount	neur. — neurology
approx. — approximately	noc. — night
ant. — anterior	N.P.O. — nothing by mouth
b.i.d. — two times a day	NS — normal saline
BM — bowel movement	O — oxygen
BP — blood pressure	OB. — obstetrics
BRP — bathroom privileges	O.D. — right eye
C — carbon	OOB — out of bed
C. — centigrade	O.S. — left eye
c — with	O.U. — both eyes
Ca — calcium	oz. — ounce
Cal. — calorie	P — phosphorous
caps. — capsules	p.c. — after meals
cc — cubic centimeter	Ped. — pediatrics
Cl — chlorine	per — by or through
CNS — central nervous system	PO or p.o. — by mouth
CBS — chronic brain syndrome	post. — posterior
c/o — complaints of	p.r.n. — whenever necessary
Cu — copper	Pt. — patient
DC — discontinue	PT — physical therapy
dr. — dram	q.d. — every day
etiol. — etiology	q.h. — every hour
ext. — exterior, external	q.i.d. — four times a day
ER — emergency room	q.s. — quantity sufficient or as
elix. — elixir	much as is required
F. — fahrenheit	S — sulfur
Fe. — iron	s — without
GI — gastrointestinal	sp. gr. — specific gravity
Gm. or gm. — gram	ss — a half
GU — genitourinary	sig. — give with the following
gr. — grain	directions
Gtt. or gtt. — drop	s.o.s. — if necessary (means
H — hydrogen	for one dose only)
(H) — hypo	stat. — immediately
H_2O — water	s.c. — subcutaneously
I — iodine	t.i.d. — three times a day
ICU — intensive care unit	TPR — temperature, pulse,
I.M. — intramuscular	respiration
inf. — inferior	tr., tinct. — tincture
int. — interior, internal	tsp. — teaspoon
I.V. — intravenous	tbl. — tablespoon
K — potassium	ung. — ointment
l. or L. — liter	Via. — by way of
lat. — lateral	V.D. — veneral disease
lb. — pound	WBC — white blood cell count

Conversion Rules

Conversion of Metric and Apothecaries' Units

1. To convert grams to grains (or milliliters to minims), multiply the number of grams (or milliliters) by 15.
   Example: change 30 grams to grains   30 x 15 = 450 grains
2. To convert grains to grams, divide the number of grains by 15 (or multiply by 0.065).
   Example: change 60 grains to grams   60 ÷ 15 = 3 grams
3. To convert grams to milligrams, move the decimal point of the grams three places to the right.
   Example: 0.250 grams = 250 milligrams
4. To convert milligrams to grams, move the decimal point of the milligrams three places to the left.
   Example: 300 milligrams = 0.3 grams

Conversion Factors for Temperature

Given	Multiply by	To Find
Fahrenheit temperature	5/9 (after subtracting 32)	Celsius temperature
Celsius temperature	9/5 (then add 32)	Fahrenheit temperature

Common Metric Prefixes

milli	one one thousandth	abbreviated as m	.001
centi	one one hundredth	abbreviated as c	.01
deci	one tenth		.1
	one		1.00
deka	ten		10.00
hecto	one hundred		100.00
kilo	one thousand	abbreviated as k	1,000.00

less than one (top 3)   more than one (bottom 3)

Metric Vocabulary

describe length or distance
   millimeter
   centimeter

describe volume
   milliliter
   liter

describe weight
   milligram
   gram
   kilogram

describe temperature
   degree Celcius (formerly Centigrade)

Metric Abbreviations

gram: a measurement of weight abbreviated as *g*
meter: a measurement of length abbreviated as *m*
liter: a measurement of volume abbreviated as *l*

Equivalence Table

Medications are measured in units of the metric system or the apothecaries' system. The following tables are approximate equivalents, but these approximate dose equivalents have the approval of the federal government's Food and Drug Administration.

A milliliter (ml) is the approximate equivalent of a cubic centimeter (cc).

Liquid Measure

Metric		Approximate Apothecaries' Equivalent
1000	ml = 1	quart
750	ml = 1½	pints
500	ml = 1	pint
250	ml = 8	fluid ounces
200	ml = 7	fluid ounces
100	ml = 3½	fluid ounces
50	ml = 1¾	fluid ounces
30	ml = 1	fluid ounce
15	ml = 4	fluid drams
10	ml = 2½	fluid drams
8	ml = 2	fluid drams
5	ml = 1¼	fluid drams
4	ml = 1	fluid dram
3	ml = 45	minims
2	ml = 30	minims
1	ml = 15	minims
0.75	ml = 12	minims
0.6	ml = 10	minims

Weight

Metric		Approximate Apothecaries' Equivalent
30	g = 1	ounce
15	g = 4	drams
10	g = 2½	drams
7.5	g = 2	drams
6	g = 90	grains
5	g = 75	grains
4	g = 60	grains (1 dram)
3	g = 45	grains
2	g = 30	grains (½ dram)
1.5	g = 22	grains
1	g = 15	grains
0.75	g = 12	grains
0.6	g = 10	grains
0.5	g = 7½	grains
0.4	g = 6	grains
0.3	g = 5	grains
0.25	g = 4	grains
0.2	g = 3	grains
0.15	g = 2½	grains
0.125	g = 2	grains
0.1	g = 1½	grains
75	mg = 1¼	grains
60	mg = 1	grain
50	mg = ¾	grain
40	mg = ⅔	grain
30	mg = ½	grain
25	mg = 3/8	grain
20	mg = ⅓	grain
15	mg = ¼	grain
12	mg = 1/5	grain
10	mg = 1/6	grain
8	mg = 1/8	grain
6	mg = 1/10	grain

Measures and Weights: Approximate Equivalents

60 gtt = 1 teaspoon = 4 cc or ml
4 cc = 60 minims
60 minims = 60 grains
60 grains = 1 dram
1 dram = 1/8 ounce
30 cc = 1 ounce
15 cc = 1 tablespoon

Houshold Measures and Weights

1 teaspoon = 1 dram
4 teaspoons = 1 tablespoon
1 tablespoon = 4 drams

Index